ACKNOWLEDGMENTS

I would like to thank the five people who contributed to the photographs and a day of fun: Susan Amer who did a great job with hair and makeup; weight specialist Donna Pickering who supervised my body positions; Angela Miller, president of The Miller Press, who coordinated us all; and, of course, Paul Schneck, master photographer. My friend Nick Stringas, Manager of the Waterside Health Club, supplied the benches and weights. You were a super crew!

My haircut is by Joseph Peragine of Elizabeth Arden.

Thanks to Andrew Irsay, weight instructor at the Vertical Club, and to Monica Mercedes, Andy's assistant, who gave me many useful suggestions for my personal weight-training program.

To my dear friend Melanie Radley, an accomplished weight lifter who was a great buddy at our Friday-night weight-lifting sessions. You added to the fun.

Thanks to Sarah Jane Freymann, my literary agent, for her confidence.

I'd like to thank Dr. Christine Wells of Arizona State University, a 1983 recipient of the Wonder Woman Award, and a friend and colleague who specializes in exercise physiology, for her thoughtful comments on the manuscript.

Finally, I'd like to express appreciation to my students and to Ellen Sue Pace, Dawn MacDonald, and other colleagues too numerous to mention.

DEDICATION

To Jerry who has encouraged me to follow my dreams.

To my Mom who has just retired from teaching English. You showed me the way!

To my son Stephen who has been waiting patiently for a book by his Mom.

To my Dad, the explorer, who taught me to strive—forever.

To Angela Miller, my editor, friend, and mentor, whose ideas and guidance made this book possible.

Thanks, everyone, for the sharing!

D1597116

CONTENTS

INTRODUCTION

Part I

Part II

Part III

Introduction

This weight-training program results from my personal weight-training experience and courses I teach at Brooklyn College. One is an activity course in physical conditioning; the other is a lecture course on the principles and theory of physical fitness in which students learn to develop individualized fitness programs.

The men in both courses tend to be knowledgeable about weight training. The women know less about it and approach it with trepidation. This book is designed to give women the courage, the knowledge, and the motivation to become physically strong.

The ideal way to become knowledgeable in weight training is by combining textual information with supervised practice. There are many weight-training books on the market for men (see the Suggested Readings at the end of this book). Since weight training is a relatively new endeavor for many women, there are fewer books to guide them in developing their own programs. And while they can use the same books as men, these are usually inappropriate. Most women are interested in body shaping and toning rather than developing the large muscles as do male body builders, and thus women find the pictures and procedures for men totally unsuitable. Even if the reader would like to begin weight training, she might be discouraged after reading a book written expressly for men.

Therefore, this introductory book provides women novices with the information and encouragement needed to begin and then maintain their own weight-training programs. Since this is a program that I have developed over the past ten years for my students and for myself, I know that it works. Weight training does such magnificent things (that's me in the pictures and I'm 42) that I plan to train with weights for the rest of my life.

The new interest in optimal well-being and physical fitness has given women the impetus to develop their physical potential. Physical-education courses at Brooklyn College are no longer required for graduation as they were in the past. However, class enrollment has not declined—it has nearly tripled. The proportion of women to men has increased dramatically.

I welcome this change. Women are there by choice, eager for knowledge, and wanting to improve their skills. They want to learn. A new age in physical fitness is dawning. This book is for all women who want to take part.

PART I
The Advantage of Weights

1
ATALANTA AWAKENS:

The Dawning of a New Ideal of Beauty—and Health

There's a new ideal image of feminine beauty. I am sure you have noticed her. She has graced the front cover of *Time* magazine in a leotard and tights. The new beauty is still lean, but also athletic, strong, energetic, and powerful. For the first time in years, women are encouraged to develop muscles, strength, and power. Actresses and TV personalities such as Jane Fonda, Linda Evans, Victoria Principal, and Raquel Welch are serious exercisers! The new image of beauty is exciting and desirable because it is combined with health, vitality, and self-confidence. Women are seeking a healthy, muscular leanness. Weight training is the fastest, easiest, and most successful way to attain this look.

It's difficult to say that a strong, muscular appearance for women is not only acceptable, but desirable, because beauty is such an individualized preference. I am sure that some men and women still find a soft, plump figure characterized by Dolly Parton pleasing. However, the fashion models who seem to set the trends in beauty have become slightly heavier than they were ten years ago and certainly more muscular, as indicated by their visible muscle definition.

In addition to the fashion messages, the fitness boom encourages women to exercise regularly, regardless of whether it is to lose weight, look their best, do something especially for themselves, experience the psychological benefits, or achieve strength in a new area. The intense interest in fitness fashions a new social group—the fit elite. Women and men who have magnificent bodies exercise at least an hour a day in stylish health clubs, pay close attention to their fitness attire, and are sexually attracted to people who are physically fit.

By exercising, many things become possible—even staying young. Jane Fonda looked superbly fit as she appeared in a bikini at the age of forty-four in her movie *On Golden Pond*. With the great success of *Jane Fonda's Workout Book,* the accompanying *Workout* cassettes and videotapes, and her new fitness salons, Jane Fonda is the celebrity fitness leader. Raquel Welch also personifies the age-retardant properties of exercise. At the age of forty-one, she created a sensation on Broadway, graced the cover of *Life* magazine, married a man considerably younger than herself, and became newly pregnant. Linda Evans, the television star of "Dynasty," has a gorgeous face and figure, just turned forty in 1983, and wrote the best-selling *Linda Evans Beauty and Exercise Book*. She appears on the front cover holding a chrome-plated dumbbell. She looks sexy, beautiful, and strong. The message is clear. You can stay young, vibrant, and beautiful by exercising.

The dawning of a new ideal in beauty and health is here! Although you have inherited a particular body type, working out with free weights will help you realize your own beauty potential, unleash a secret store of energy, and increase your self-confidence.

If you want a beautiful body, you must exercise. Regardless of your genetic inheritance, whether you are too heavy, too thin, or have a super body, you will look better if you work out. Physical endowment, just like any other inherited capability, such as musical talent or artistic ability, will not mature without training.

You can get into shape fast with free weights. Whether you are going on a cruise, reporting for a modeling assignment, making an important appearance in a bathing suit, or training for a sport activity, weight training is the most successful, nonsurgical way to develop the firmest, leanest, and strongest body that you can have in the least amount of time.

It is amazing how quickly you can build a firm, rounded bust, taut torso, a firm waist, and a flat abdomen. With weights, you also can reduce the flab on your upper arms and tone your thighs and calves. Start on your weight training program today and discover what an ego boost it can be.

"Weight training" is an all-inclusive term that refers to any exercise that includes the use of weights or added resistance. You might be using Nautilus or Universal weight machines, dumbbells (the small, hand-held weights generally used in pairs), a barbell (the long bar with various weights on each end), or a variety of gadgets. "Free weight" refers specifically to dumbbells and barbells. You are "free" to move them in a multitude of different ways.

Both free weights and the weight machines have distinct advantages and disadvantages. It's impossible to say that one is better than the other—even in the development of muscle. Nautilus enthusiasts swear by the Nautilus; free-weight users claim barbells produce the fastest, most pronounced physical changes. Clearly both are successful approaches to body toning and shaping.

Free weights are the focus of this book because they are inexpensive, easily stored at home, and enable you to work out whenever you have fifteen to twenty minutes available. Of course, if you prefer the sociability and additional facilities of a health club, these routines can be done in a weight room. I prefer a combination of exercising at home and at a health club. Sometimes I work out when I watch TV; at other times, I simply need to get out of my apartment. The important thing is to experiment and see what's right for you.

Weight training will not cause you to develop the bulky, stereotyped muscles of women Olympic-caliber shot-putters. These women are successful in such strength-dependent sports because they were *born* with a genetic predisposition toward large muscles. Their naturally occurring high levels of steroids, their body proportions, and natural muscle length enable them to develop unusually bulky muscles. I have been weight training for the past ten years. I still have the long, slim muscles that I've always had. The weight-training program gives me more shapely and more defined muscles, gets rid of flab, and creates new energy. The average woman, like you and me, cannot develop the physique of a champion body builder regardless of how many hours a day she trains!

Try this weight routine for a few weeks and test the results for yourself. One particularly reassuring point to keep in mind is that muscles don't appear overnight. In fact, competitive body builders work out six to eight hours a day. If you find that you are one of the infinitesimal number of women who are prone to large muscles and that you are developing larger muscles than you would like, simply exercise a little less than you have been doing. They'll disappear.

2
Muscle Strength

In addition to giving you a wondrous body, weight training enhances your health. "Health" no longer denotes a mere absence of disease; it refers to a high level of physical functioning or wellness. A few of the benefits that accrue from weight training are better posture, weight loss, lower blood pressure, greater glucose tolerance, and the prevention of diabetes mellitus in adults, an increase in high-density lipoproteins which are negatively correlated with heart disease, increased coronary efficiency, a reduction of menstrual pain, minimalization of complications during pregnancy and delivery, and probably the prevention of osteoporosis which is prevalent in older women.

Weight training is especially important if you have back problems. Performed properly, weight training alleviates whatever back problems that you may have and helps prevent them if you have encountered no problems.

Much back pain is of neuromuscular origin and reflects your general stress level. Weight training is a marvelous stress-reduction technique. You concentrate on something other than your daily problems, get rid of pent-up energy, and prepare for another day by strengthening your body. You might consider weight training as preparing your body for combat. By developing strong back and abdominal muscles, you are much less prone to muscle spasms resulting from stress.

If your back problems are structural and your physician has indicated that you have a degenerating disc, again it is helpful to strengthen the surrounding muscles. In general, the stronger your back and abdominal muscles, the less strain there is on your vertebrae. Since you must take care not to place additional strain on your weakened back, a special, gentle set of exercises is suggested in this book.

The health benefits of exercise are so important that a noted physician and back specialist, Dr. Hans Kraus, coined the phrase "hypokinetic disease" to refer to the multitude of ailments that result from too little exercise.

Muscular strength, your primary gain in any weight routine, gives you the ability to physically complete your daily activities and to use a smaller proportion of the total amount of strength that you have available. Thus, you are less taxed as you carry the groceries, walk to the bus, and climb the stairs and have considerably more energy when you arrive home. You'll find this benefit one of the most important reasons for exercising. You no longer will be so tired at the end of the day that you are forced to sit in a chair and watch TV. Rather than your free-weight program taking time from your day, it literally will give you added hours.

In addition to physical health, muscle strength will, believe it or not, enhance your psychological well-being. It definitely improves your self-concept, body awareness, and self-esteem. As you experience the physical improvements, note your willingness to stick with the program, and observe the increasing ease of the exercises. (If you are especially interested in the influence of exercise on self-concept, refer to my chapter "Running Toward Psychological Well-Being," which reviews the latest research in the area and is listed in the Suggested Readings.)

Whether weight training, like running, influences other psychological characteristics such as your on-going level of depression, anxiety, vigor, and fatigue is not known. I simply am not aware of a single research study on the psychological effects of weight training. A recent study by

Dr. David Owen and myself did indicate, however, that the effects of swimming were comparable to those of running (Berger and Owen, 1983). Swimmers were significantly less tense, depressed, angry, and confused and were more invigorated after exercising than before. Whether weight training would have the same results is unclear, because running and swimming are more aerobic than a free-weight routine. We definitely need additional research before we will understand the psychological benefits of weight training. Such research is important because of its implications for mental health and the ease with which a free-weight routine can be included in a woman's life.

To summarize, a free-weight routine is the best way—without a doubt—to firm, tone, and shape your body. It definitely promotes a higher level of well-being and probably enhances your psychological outlook. If you are interested in developing cardiovascular fitness in addition to strength, increase the number of repetitions and use lighter weights. Activities such as jogging, biking, and swimming are ideal ways to supplement your free-weight workout.

3
Why Weight Training Is a Must Supplement for All Sports

An old adage in sports that makes a lot of sense is that you condition yourself to play a sport. You don't play a sport to get into condition. What this means is that if you are not physically fit, you will not be able to perform up to your capabilities in a particular sport and that the likelihood of injury will be high. In most sports such as tennis, gymnastics, and swimming, trying to get into condition by playing the sport itself will take you much longer than will a more concentrated strength-and-endurance program. This is particularly true early in the season when you tend to be less fit.

You need a weight-training program to maximize your sport skills, whether you are participating on a recreational or competitive level. Weight training, however, is not equally important in each activity. Sports can be categorized according to the importance of weight training. The primary categories are as follows:

(1) *Those for whom weight training is a must.* These sports require muscle strength and are represented by gymnastics, softball, tennis, swimming, bodybuilding, and field events in track.

(2) *Those that employ primarily the lower part of the body and aesthetically need a supplemental weight-training program to effect a more balanced upper-body physique.* Running, bicycling, skating, skiing, and dance illustrate this need.

(3) *Those sports for which a weight-training program seems less important, but still would benefit from*

some additional conditioning. Basketball, dance, diving, and volleyball fall into this category.

Although my generalized free-weight program is useful for competitors in *all* sports, a specific program designed for a particular sport would be even better. Devise your own program by following my suggestions in Part II and the following principles.

Muscle Specificity

Changes in muscle strength and endurance occur only in those muscles which are being used. Thus, if you need additional upper-arm strength, be sure to concentrate on these muscles.

Strength or Endurance

If muscle endurance is of primary importance, as in distance running or swimming, complete many repetitions (i.e., 15 to 50) with lighter weights. If you need maximum strength, as in high jumping or putting the shot, perform fewer repetitions (7 to 10) with maximum weight. Perform 10 to 15 repetitions if you need a little of both.

Specificity of Movement

The closer your weight-training movement reflects the actual sport movements, the greater the benefit of your weight training. For example, swimmers can weight-train by swimming with only their arms, and baseball players can use a weighted bat. Beyond a mid-amount of conditioning to develop strength and to prevent injury, research shows that performing the sport activity itself is probably the most productive type of practice.
Good luck in your sport endeavors!

4
Stronger Muscles
Will Help You
Be Slimmer:
They Burn More Calories

Weight training is a superb way to prevent and control obesity. The relationship between exercise and weight control is complex, and researchers are just beginning to unravel the interlocking parts. Thus, it is difficult to separate the sense from the nonsense or wishful thinking that appears in many popular magazines. To help clarify your thinking, I will briefly review some of the current research. If you'd like additional information, refer to an article on "Exercise and Obesity" by Thompson, Jarvie, Lahey, and Cureton, and to "Physical Activity in the Development and Control of Obesity" by Brownell and Stunkard, which are listed in the Suggested Readings.

To appreciate the importance of maintaining a desirable weight for health and appearance, keep in mind that overweight people have a higher incidence of cardiovascular diseases such as strokes, arteriosclerosis, hypertension, and varicose veins. In fact, susceptibility to these diseases increases 30 percent for each 10-percent increase above ideal body weight (see the article in the Suggested Readings by Jeffrey and Lemnitzer).

Weight training contributes to a desirable loss of body fat in a variety of ways. Despite the widely publicized need to perform an inhuman amount of exercise to merely lose one pound, exercise is a crucial component of any successful lifelong weight loss. Let me tell you why.

Exercise Burns More Calories

Vigorous movement clearly expends more calories than normal daily activities such as sitting at a desk, reading, washing dishes, or even scrubbing the kitchen floor. The important factors to consider when you determine the caloric cost of any exercise session are (1) *exercise intensity* (how strenuous it is as indicated by your heart rate), (2) *exercise duration* (the length of time you exercise), and (3) *exercise frequency* (the number of days per week that you exercise). A combination of these three exercise parameters determines the actual number of calories you burn. The more strenuous and more often you exercise for a given amount of time, the greater your weight loss. For example, the caloric cost per minute of running is larger than that for walking, because running is a more intense form of exercise. However, you expend the *same number of calories* whether you walk two miles or run two miles. The walking simply requires more of your time—thus you have compensated for the reduced intensity of walking by increasing the *duration* of your exercise session. The point is that you have done the same amount of *work* by walking and by running a mile and burning the same number of calories. Of course, the running is more efficient because it requires less time. Running may burn a few more calories than walking because it elevates your metabolic rate during and after exercise (see "Exercise Increases Your Basal Metabolic Rate" in this chapter).

To facilitate weight loss in your weight-training program, you can choose whether you prefer to eliminate rest periods between the exercises and thus increase the intensity of your workout, or whether to include a few breaks and spend a longer time exercising. As long as your total amount of work is the same, the caloric expenditure or weight loss will be approximately the same.

Exercise Decreases Your Appetite

Weight training also decreases your appetite. A variety of controlled studies indicates that mild to moderate exercise (between twenty minutes and one hour) has this effect. Strenuous exercise—between two and six hours in duration—increases your food intake, but not your weight. However, unless you decide to become a competitive body builder, you will not fall into the "strenuous" category with your free-weight program.

Exercise Increases Your Basal Metabolic Rate

Another way in which weight training contributes to weight loss is that it is thought to elevate your basal metabolic rate for a period far beyond your actual exercise session. It is encouraging to know that after you stop exercising, your body still burns more calories than normal. The actual length and amount of increase in metabolic rate is not clear and has been reported to range between four and forty-eight hours and to increase between 10 and 18 percent. Such changes would result in a loss of four to five pounds over a year's time.

The increase in basal metabolism is especially important if you are dieting, because dieting actually produces a 15 to 30 percent decrease in your metabolic rate! The more often you have dieted throughout your life, the faster your metabolic rate decreases and the longer it takes for it to return to baseline levels when you end caloric restriction. Regular and severe caloric restriction without exercising retards permanent weight loss. If you want to lose weight and *keep it off*, you must exercise. In the long run, exercise is a more successful and more comfortable way to lose weight and to prevent its return.

By Exercising, You Lose Fat, Not Water or Muscle

Another exciting influence of weight training on weight loss is its major effect on body composition. Exercise increases the ratio of lean to fat tissue. If you lose weight by exercising, you lose a much greater amount of fat tissue, much less lean muscle tissue, and considerably less water than if you lose the very same number of pounds from dieting.

Loss of muscle tissue in any weight-loss program is exceedingly undesirable. You need it to conduct your daily activities without undue stress, strain, and tiredness, *and* the lean muscle tissue has a much higher metabolic rate than the fat tissue. Loss of muscle tissue in any weight-loss program is self-defeating. You need its high metabolic rate in order to continue to burn energy!

Hints for Additional Weight Loss

If you are serious about losing weight in addition to toning your muscles when you weight-train, (1) plan to diet while exercising and (2) increase the amount of physical activity in your daily activities. Combining exercise with caloric restriction not only increases the speed of your weight loss, but it tends to reduce the plateau that dieters encounter when their weight stabilizes and they fail to lose additional weight. A diet that is especially effective has been developed by Dr. Peter Wood, deputy director of the Heart Disease Prevention Program at Stanford University; his book is listed in the Suggested Readings. I recommend it highly!

Try to increase your physical activity and caloric expenditure throughout the day. Walk up a flight or two of stairs rather than use the elevator. Walk a couple of blocks whenever you have the opportunity rather than drive.

The Scales Don't Always Tell the Truth!

Just because you weigh the same on the scales, don't despair! The scales do not tell all. If you work out with weights and diet for several weeks, you undoubtedly will be thinner. Muscle tissue is considerably heavier than fat. Losing several inches of fat and replacing it with a little muscle will result in a leaner appearance but not necessarily in a weight loss. The loss of fat will be observable in the way your clothes fit. In addition to the decrease in body measurements, your muscles will be firmer and more shapely. Your posture will be more upright, and your abdomen flatter. You'll look great! Keep on exercising.

PART II
Weight-Training Exercise Program

5
Amount of Exercise

It is very important to determine the right amount of exercise for you. Clearly, this varies according to your activity level at the present time. Regardless of your fitness level, your goal is to *exercise as strenuously as you can without experiencing any muscle soreness twenty-four hours later*. If you experience muscular pain the following day, reflect on the amount of exercise you did with that particular body part and then do a little less when you exercise again. Because this is a very individualized matter, you will need to experiment using the following guidelines.

Perform ten to fifteen repetitions of each exercise. Each of the ten or fifteen movements is called a repetition, or a "rep." Each group of movements is a "set." Your goal is to completely fatigue that muscle group by the end of a set. This is indicated by your inability to perform one more rep. Thus, for fifteen reps, you use a lighter weight than if you do ten reps. Decide for yourself whether you prefer to complete ten with heavy weights, or fifteen with the lighter ones.

Complete one and eventually two sets (you can rest between sets) of each exercise before starting on the next one. Rest as long as you need between sets, but do a second set before moving on to your next exercise. When you first start, you may find finishing one complete set of the exercises for each body part is too difficult. If this is so, perform only one of the exercises for each body part. Still complete the ten reps of whichever exercise you choose. Soon you will be able to complete one set for each exercise, and then two.

Your goal is to lift as much weight as you can and still complete ten to fifteen repetitions in one or two sets. When two sets become rather easy, increase the weight that you are using in order that it is again quite difficult for you to complete ten reps. *To obtain maximum benefit from each exercise, it is important to stress each muscle group to exhaustion.* In this way, you obtain maximum physical toning and development in the least amount of practice time possible. The principle is to TRAIN LESS, BUT TO WORK HARDER! The harder the exercise, the better the results!

High-intensity exercise must be brief. If you can do an exercise for a long time, the intensity is not high enough. You cannot train for both intensity and endurance simultaneously. You reach maximum intensity when you contract a muscle as much as you can at a particular moment. Your goal is to experience momentary muscular failure at the end of your tenth or twelfth repetition. This is characterized by the feeling that the last rep was difficult and that the next one is impossible. Do be careful, though, not to use such a heavy weight that you cannot perform the exercise according to the suggested form.

The general principle to follow at all times is to focus on quality of movement rather than quantity.

For the hand-held weights, start with three pounds. If these are too heavy, perform the exercises for a week or two with no weight, or with a sixteen-ounce canned product from your pantry before trying them again.

Initially for ankle weights, wear a pair of heavy shoes such as those for jogging. You can purchase a pair of two-pound ankle weights when you are ready. When your ankle weights become too light, wear both your shoes and the weights before purchasing the readily available four-pound weights.

Experiment with the number of reps and sets for variety and motivation as well as to emphasize desired results. Reduce the number of reps and increase the amount of weight. This will strengthen and contour your body most quickly. You can also hold the number of repetitions constant and increase the weight within a set. You can reduce the amount of weight and increase the number of reps. This way you can avoid boredom by changing your routines.

If you want to lose weight, reduce your caloric intake and maintain a free-weight routine. To burn more calories when you exercise, focus on a large number of repetitions (15 to 30) with reduced rest intervals to emphasize caloric expenditure. Participate in an aerobic activity such as running, biking, or swimming on alternate days to help with weight reduction. With regular exercise—and no increase in caloric intake—you will see definite firming and shaping in three to four weeks.

To build muscle and thus gain weight, focus on using heavy weights with a low number of repetitions (4 to 6 reps with the heaviest weights possible). More pronounced changes require four to six weeks.

6
Reveal Your Body

Whenever you work out with weights, wear something that reveals your body! The reason that body builders often wear tiny bikinis when they train is not that they are exhibitionists but that it is very important to be able to SEE YOUR BODY.

If you are exercising at home, put on a bikini. If you don't own one, don't worry. Just wear any bathing suit or leotard. You'll lose the impact of actually seeing the middle portion of your body, but you will still get a general impression. If you are exercising all by yourself, you could exercise in underwear or nothing at all.

If you decide to lift weights at your exercise club or gym, wear as revealing an outfit as you can. Clearly a leotard and tights are superior to shorts and a T-shirt. The tights are not necessary; they simply allow you to bend in a variety of positions without your wondering what might be showing. You can relax and concentrate on your training program.

You should also work out in front of a mirror, the larger the better. It's gratifying to see those muscles strain. You certainly feel them working, but it is encouraging to actually see them and to know all of the wonderful things that you are doing. Seeing your muscles contract and relax as you perform various movements reinforces the physical sensations and helps you develop a heightened awareness of your body. If you're wondering what area of your body is being firmed by a particular exercise, just look in the mirror. You'll see the muscles working.

Wearing a bikini clearly exposes your "trouble" spots. Be brave and take a good look at them! You don't need to expose them to the world. However, as your own exercise expert, you need to be fully aware of them. I find that being reminded of my problem areas as I work out pushes me to work harder and to focus on these spots. Free-weight training will firm the parts of your body that you now consider your least attractive assets.

I'd like to say one last thing about the advantages of wearing a bathing suit to exercise. It reminds me to cut down on what I eat. Being aware of my body is related to what I eat, and I am far less likely to snack on something that is loaded with calories.

Ask someone to take a picture of you in a bathing suit before you start your weight-training program and then at regular intervals (a recommended period is every month) to record your results. It will be exciting to see your success, and you will be able to assess your progress objectively.

7
Breathing

Some weight lifters emphasize the importance of breathing in and out at specific times during an exercise. I think that this makes exercising unduly complicated and clutters your mind with unnecessary detail. Since I would like you to concentrate on the feeling in the muscles that you are exercising rather than on breathing, I have one general suggestion. EXHALE DURING THE MOST DIFFICULT PORTION OF THE MOVEMENT; INHALE DURING THE EASIER HALF. I don't know exactly why, but exhaling seems to make the difficult portion less taxing. It is no catastrophe, however, if you breathe in and out at the "wrong" time.

THE IMPORTANT THING IS TO *BREATHE*! Holding your breath elevates your blood pressure and tends to decrease your strength and thus the intensity of your workout. With a bit of practice, breathing will come naturally. If you find that it helps, exhale during the more difficult portion of the exercise.

8
Abdominal and Lower-Back Exercises

Your abdominal and lower-back muscles work as a team. One set of muscles contracts for the first half of the movement and the other set then contracts to bring you back to the starting position. For example, contracting your abdominals brings your head to your knees; contracting your lower back returns you to an upright position. Because of this complementary action, exercises designed expressly to strengthen your abdominal muscles generally strengthen your lower back and vice versa.

Of all the muscles in your body, your abdominals require the greatest amount of work to keep in shape. Competitive body builders who otherwise exercise on alternate days exercise their abdominals daily. If body builders who have firm, flat abdominals find it necessary to focus on this set of muscles, then you and I should give them daily attention too.

A weight-training program for the mid-portion of your body is, without a doubt, the best way to firm and tone these muscles. In the normal course of a day, we rarely use our abdominal, waist, hip, and buttock muscles, thus they are the first ones to become flaccid. Even if we participate in specific sport activities such as swimming, jogging, and tennis, we still do not give the middle portions of our bodies a workout. Unless you are genetically blessed with a super-flat abdomen, and I do not know many women who are, you definitely need a weight-training program for this portion of your body. It will work wonders.

Begin every weight-training session with abdominal exercises. They're great for warming up and for getting you into a hard-working frame of mind. Do not save them for the end. You'll be too tired to do a decent job for this important area.

When you first begin, try to complete one set of 10 to 12 reps. When you're able, complete 2 sets. Feel free to include as many as 15 reps in each set. However, unless you are on an unusually serious weight-reducing program, do not perform more than 15. If you wish to increase the difficulty of the movement, use additional weight and follow the general guidelines of 10 to 12 reps and 1 to 2 sets.

A real bonus in doing abdominal and lower-back exercises is that it is great preventive medicine for future back problems.

If you are feeling energetic, repeat your abdominal exercises at the end of your workout for double duty.

Tips:

- To relax your abdominals after exercising: Lie with your back flat on the floor and hug your knees to your chest.
- If you wish to lose weight, especially fat, in addition to firming, be sure to exercise *and diet*.

CRUNCHES

Goal:

To tone the lower and upper abdominal region, primarily the rectus abdominis, one of the largest muscles in your

15 to 30

1 to 2 sets

Redo at end
of session

body. I find that this is a very important exercise because it is one of the few that truly focuses on that very problematic region between your waist and pubis bone, your lower abdominal area.

Equipment:

A weight bench or chair, and a 5- to 8-pound hand weight for the advanced level.

Amount:

10 to 15 reps; 1 to 2 sets

Instructions:

1. Lie on the floor with your back flat against it. Rest your lower legs on the bench so that your thighs are perpendicular to the floor. (Fig. Ab1)

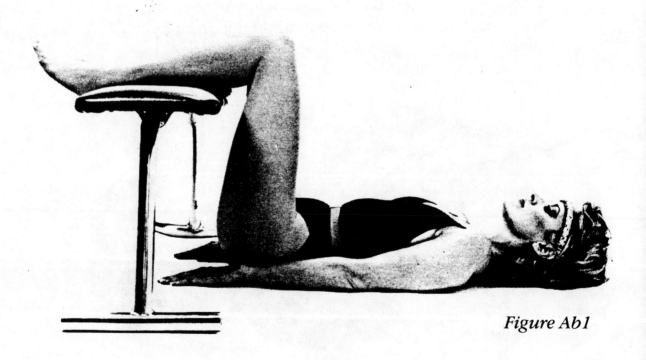

Figure Ab1

2. In a *slow* sustained movement, simultaneously
   • Round head and shoulders toward center of your body.
   • Raise hips high off the floor toward shoulders.
   • Forcefully exhale. (Fig. Ab2)

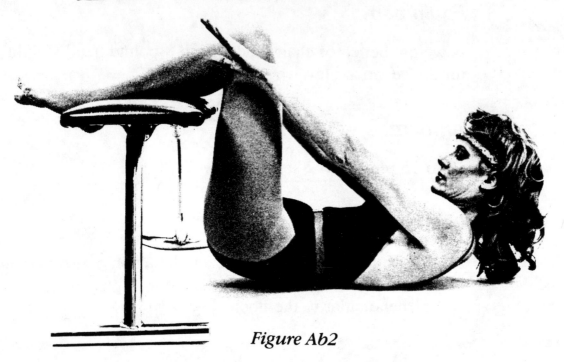

Figure Ab2

3. Vary your arm placement to increase the difficulty.
   • Beginning position: Extend your hands in front of your shoulders. Whatever you do, <u>do not</u> cheat by <u>swinging your arms</u>. Note <u>how high my derriere is off the floor</u>. (Fig. Ab3)

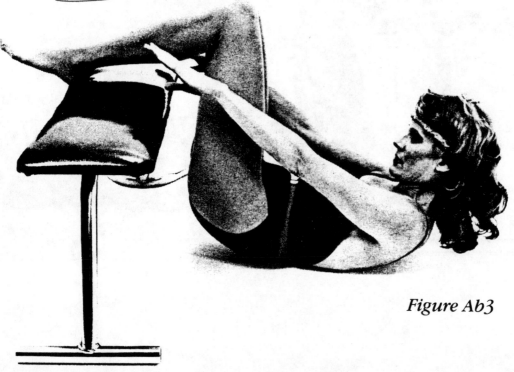

Figure Ab3

- Intermediate position: Clasp your hands behind your head with your elbows out at the side.
- Advanced position: Hold a weight in front of your chest. (Fig. Ab4)

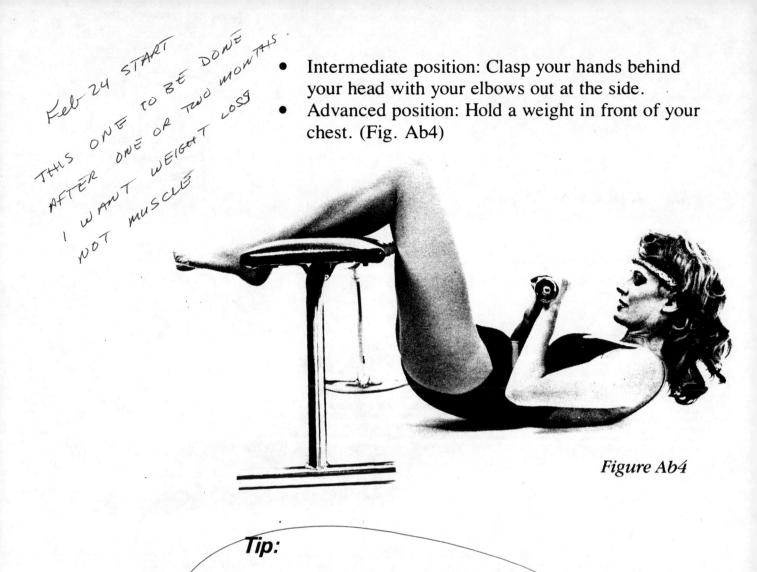

Figure Ab4

Tip:

- Avoid "jerking" to get up.

FLAT BACK BICYCLE

Goal:

Upper and lower abdominals, serratus anterior, erector spinae, and quadriceps are the primary muscles that you will firm.

Equipment:

None for the beginning level; 2-pound ankle weights, if you are more advanced; bench.

Amount:

10 to 15 reps; 1 to 2 sets

FLASH!
Quality is more
important than
quantity!

Instructions:

1. The starting position: Lie flat on the bench or floor with your left leg extended and your right leg tucked to your chest. Your hands are at your side. (Fig. Ab5)

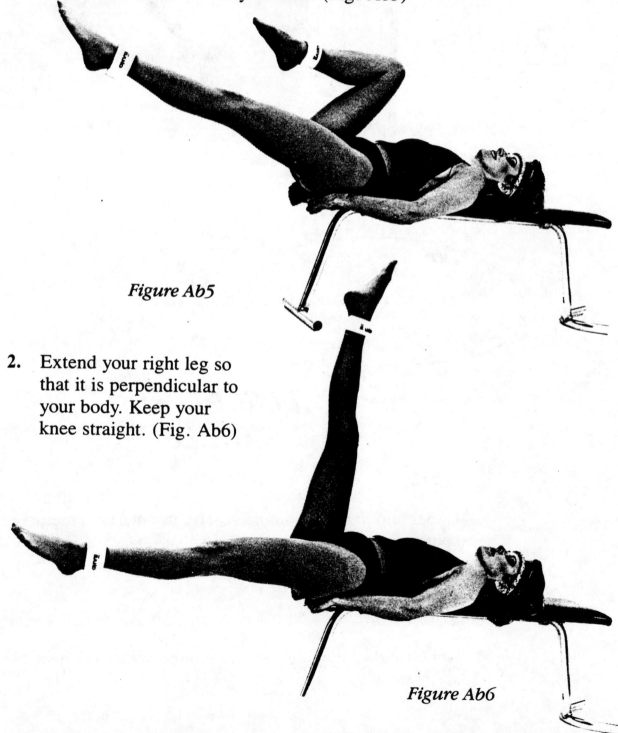

Figure Ab5

2. Extend your right leg so that it is perpendicular to your body. Keep your knee straight. (Fig. Ab6)

Figure Ab6

3. Slowly lower that leg to the floor and simultaneously raise your left knee to your chest just as though you were riding a bicycle. Avoid touching the floor with your feet. (Figs. Ab7 and Ab8)

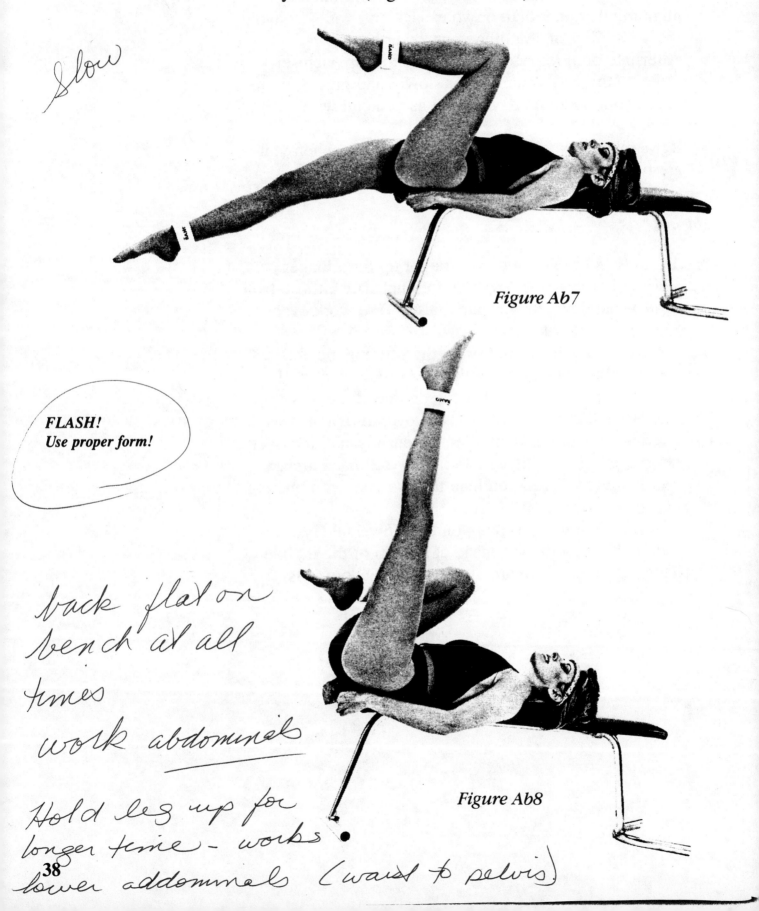

slow

Figure Ab7

FLASH!
Use proper form!

*back flat on
bench at all
times*

work abdominals

Figure Ab8

*Hold leg up for
longer time - works
lower abdominals (waist to pelvis)*

38

Tips:

- Concentrate on keeping your lower back on the bench or floor at all times. This focuses the work on your abdominals rather than on your back and you will avoid the possibility of straining your lower back.
- Alternate pointing and flexing your toes in each set.
- Execute this movement rather slowly and gracefully to stress your abdominals as much as you can with each cycle.
- Remember to hug your knees to your chest when you are finished with your abdominals.

back on bench

Variations:

1. Holding your extended leg straight up for a longer period requires your lower abdominals (i.e., those from your waist down rather than waist up) to work even harder. Go for it!

2. As you build abdominal strength, you may be able to move both legs together rather than individually. (I'm not up to this one myself. I'm convinced that if you have long legs in relation to your overall height, this exercise is more difficult than if your legs are relatively short). If you try this variation and your back arches and leaves the floor, continue the exercise with one leg at a time.

3. You may like to try it lying on the Universal Gym incline board with your head at the top of the incline. This puts even more pressure on your abdominals.

Special Abdominal and Back Exercises for Women Who Already Have Experienced Serious Back Problems

If you have problems with your lower back, substitute the following two exercises for the Crunches and Flat Back Bicycle. The Squeeze and the Cat are not very taxing and do quite a good job at toning. You need no equipment for either of these gentle exercises.

Feel free to do these exercises if your back is fine and you simply want more abdominal work. However, if you have no back problems, do not cheat by doing the Squeeze and the Cat instead of the Crunches and the Flat Back Bicycle. They should be additions rather than substitutions.

THE SQUEEZE

Goal:

To strengthen and tone abdominals and lower back. This gentle exercise primarily uses the rectus abdominis and erector spinae muscles.

Amount:

10 to 15 reps; 1 to 2 sets

Instructions:

1. Lie flat on the floor, knees bent, arms stretched out. (Fig. Ab9)
2. Contract your abdominals and push your lower back as flat against the floor as possible. Hold for a full 5 seconds. (Fig. Ab10)
3. Contract your abdominals and raise your lower back to a moderate arch. (Fig. A11)
4. Relax for a moment and try it again.

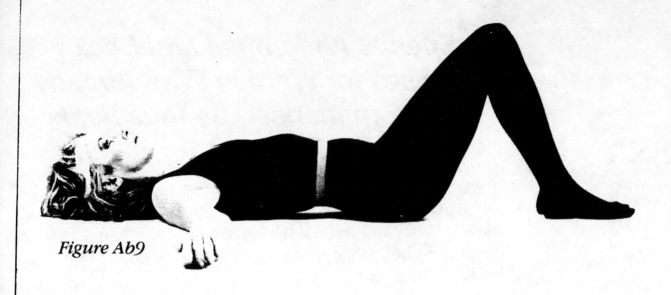

Figure Ab9

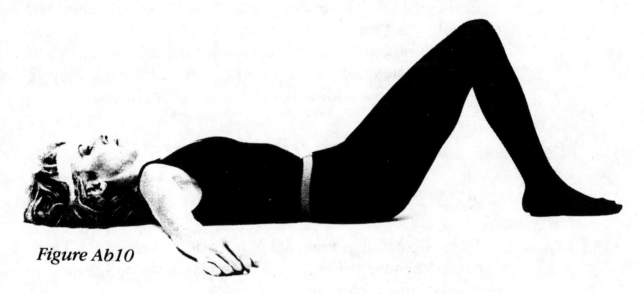

Figure Ab10

FLASH!
Focus on eliminating all of the space between you and the floor!

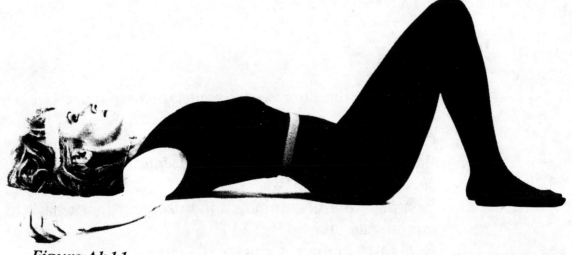

Figure Ab11

41

THE CAT

Goal:

The wide variety of muscle groups in this exercise include the ones of principal interest, namely, the rectus abdominis and erector spinae as well as the serratus anterior, latissimus dorsi, and trapezius.

Amount:

10 to 15 reps; 1 to 2 sets

Instructions:

1. Starting position: Palms and knees are on the floor. (Fig. Ab12)
    *   Hands are directly under your shoulders.
    *   Knees are directly under your hips.
    *   Your back is perfectly straight.

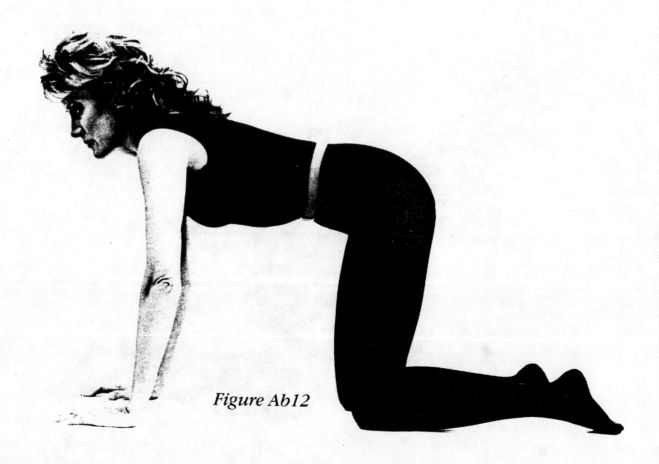

Figure Ab12

2. Round your back as high as possible, tuck your chin to your chest, and contract your abdominals. (Fig. Ab13)

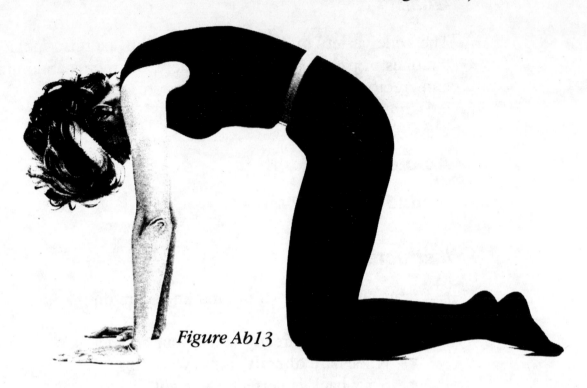

Figure Ab13

3. Slowly reverse the movement by raising your chin and arching your back. (Fig. Ab14)

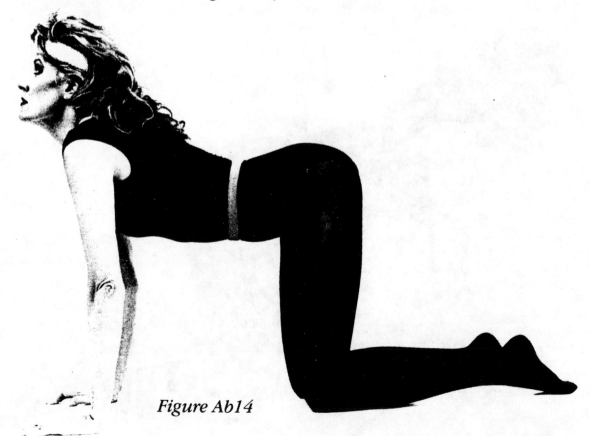

Figure Ab14

Tips:

- Start with your coccyx as you begin to round your back. When you reverse the movement, raise your chin and begin to arch your shoulders, then your waist and hips simultaneously.
- As you flex and extend your back, focus on moving it vertebra by vertebra.

At end

lie on back flat
hug knees to chest

9
BUST

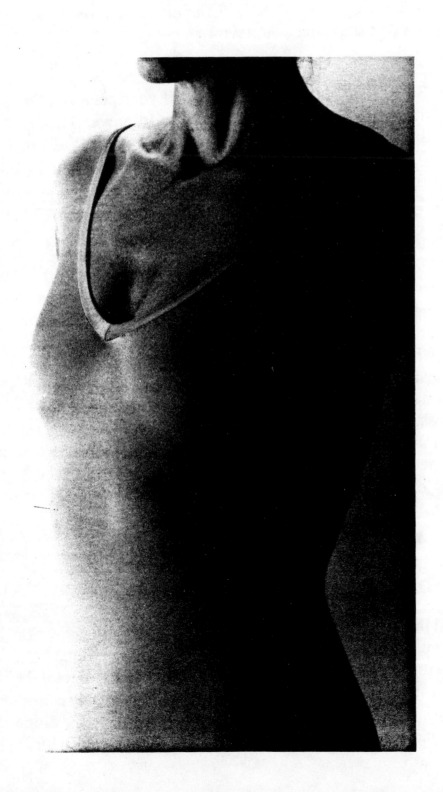

Exercise will not give you the super-large bust advertised i
the classified sections of the magazines. In fact, unless you
have inherited a tendency for large breasts, nothing, excep
plastic surgery, gaining a huge amount of weight, or
becoming pregnant, will do that for you. If you are
convinced that you would be much happier with larger
breasts, I recommend plastic surgery. Several of my friend
have had the operation and are quite happy with the results
What exercise will do is firm and make more definite the
breast tissue that you have.

Bust exercises that firm and build your pectoralis major
muscles are particularly important in preventing the sagging
that results naturally from the downward pull of gravity. If
you have large breasts, or if you are past the age of thirty,
give special attention to the following exercises in order to
reduce the sagging you most likely will encounter.

I recommend you always wear a supportive bra (in contrast
to one that is either flimsy or worn out) if you wear a cup
size that is "A" or larger. If you are concerned about your
breasts eventually drooping, prevent them from bouncing
while you exercise. You do not need an expensive bra
especially designed for exercise. What you do need is one
that is supportive and comfortable and that does not have
elastic straps. Elastic straps wear out quickly and permit
too much breast movement. There are many bras available
that are more attractive and less expensive than the special
"exercise bras."

DUMBBELL PRESS

Goal:

This is considered a "basic" rather than an "isolation"
exercise because it employs many muscle groups. The
DUMBBELL PRESS firms and builds your pectoral and
deltoid muscles which flex your upper arm. A secondary
focus is firming the latissimus dorsi, the muscle along the
side of your back which extends all the way to your

trapezius. This muscle gives body builders their V-shaped backs and is employed to extend your upper arm. Firming it decreases the loose skin that accumulates at the top and bottom of your bra. This exercise also requires you to use your triceps and deltoids.

Equipment:

Relatively heavy free weights (you can probably handle 8 to 10 pounds) and a flat bench.

Amount:

10 to 15 reps; 1 to 2 sets

Instructions:

1. Lie on a flat bench with your knees up and feet resting on the end of the bench. Keep your lower back flat against the bench while you work. Hold a pair of heavier-than-usual dumbbells directly above your shoulders with your arms extended. The dumbbells should be parallel to your body.
(Figs. B1 and B2)

Slow

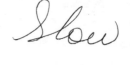

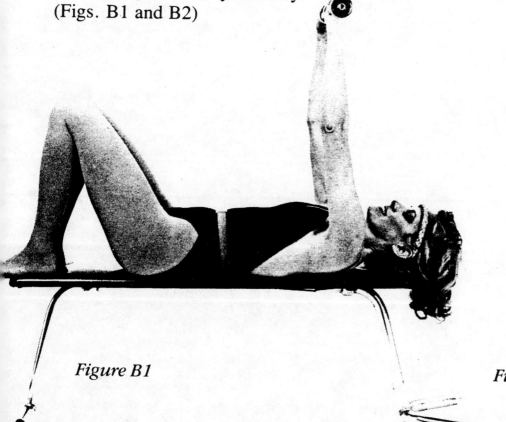

Figure B1

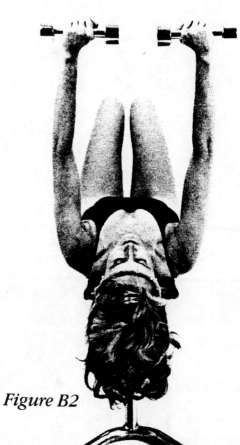

Figure B2

2. Lower the dumbbells VERY SLOWLY so that each repetition really counts. (Fig. B3)
3. As you lower the dumbbells, lower your elbows as far as possible for *maximum stretching of the "pects,"* which encourages the most rapid development of your pects. (Figs. B4 and B5)

Tip:

• This exercise is quite useful as a warm-up for the ones that follow. It prevents the likelihood of injury to your shoulder which is one of your weakest joints.

Variation:

If you don't have a bench, perform this same exercise while standing. The only disadvantage to this position is that it does not stress your pects as much as when you are lying on the bench, and focuses more on the deltoids and triceps. Of course, you still are employing your pectorals. Your trapezius is a secondary focus of the standing dumbbell press, and your lower-back, abdominal, and leg muscles serve as stabilizers.

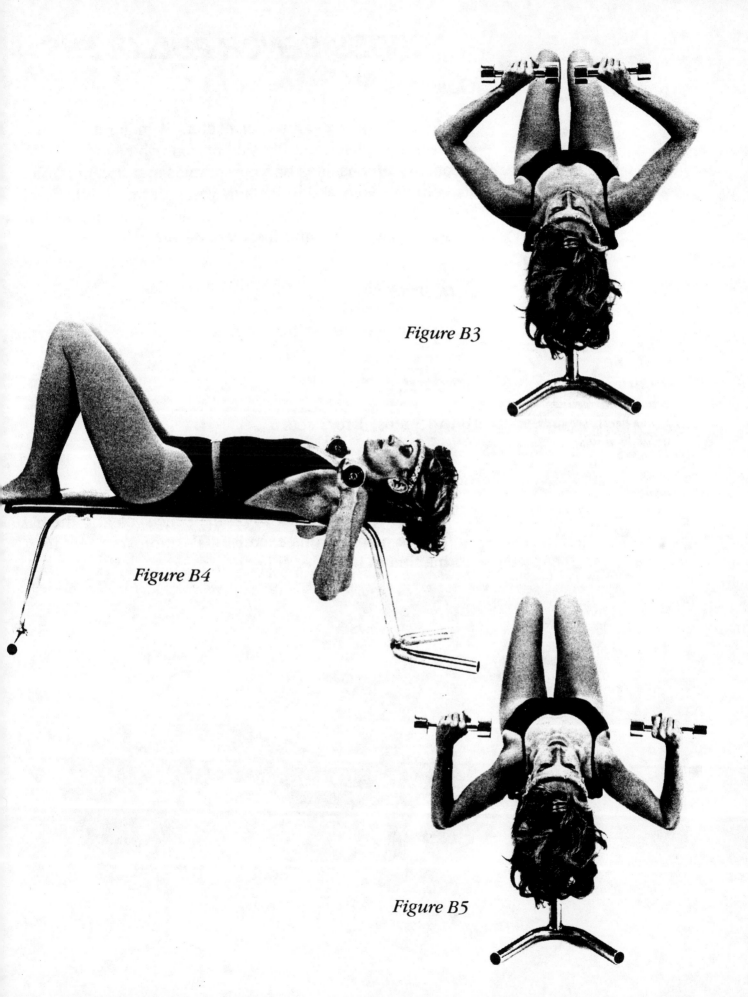

Figure B3

Figure B4

Figure B5

49

CROSS-BENCH PULLOVERS

Goal:

This exercise is great for your pectoralis major and minor and serratus muscles at the side of your rib cage. A secondary emphasis is on your deltoids and triceps. You also employ your abdominals as you pull the weight from above your head down to your shoulders. It is one of my favorites. The stretching feels wonderful.

Equipment:

Flat bench and hand-held weights.

FLASH!
Focus on the feeling in your pects, serratus, and abdominals!

Amount:

10 to 15 reps; 1 to 2 sets

Instructions:

1. Shoulders rest crosswise on the bench (clearly the basis for the name of this exercise). Position your feet for maximum balance. (Fig. B6)

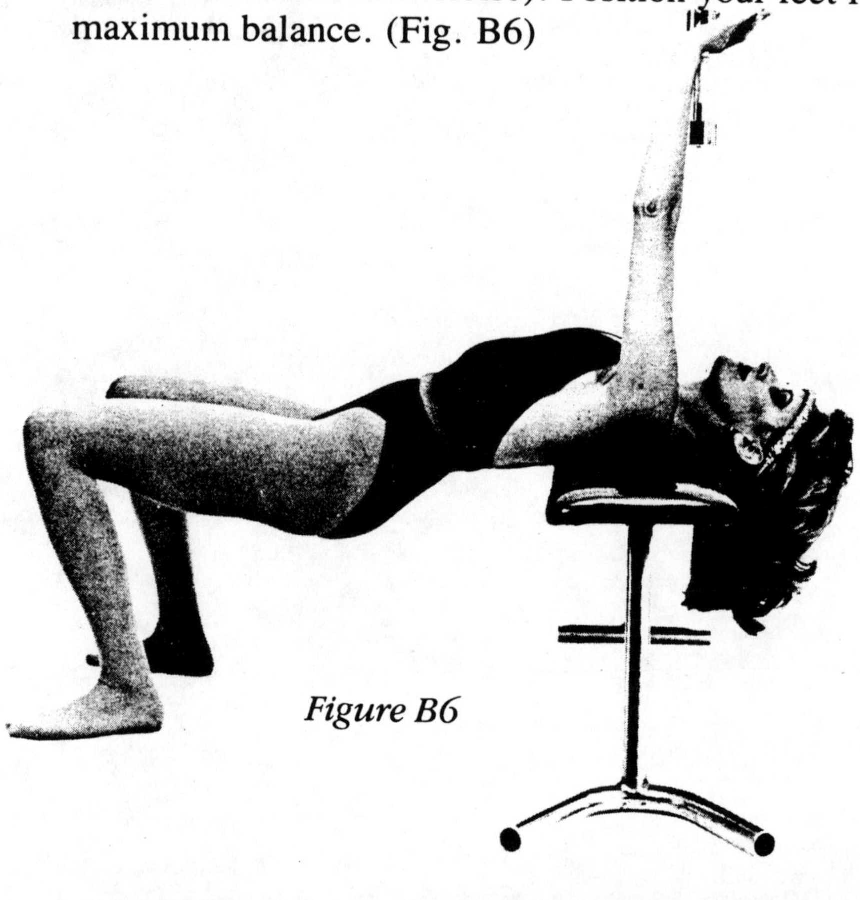

Figure B6

2. Wrap your thumbs around the single, heavy weight. Make a triangle with each thumb forming two sides and the fingers of each hand forming the other two sides (Fig. B7). This "hole" catches the top of the weight. (Fig. B8)

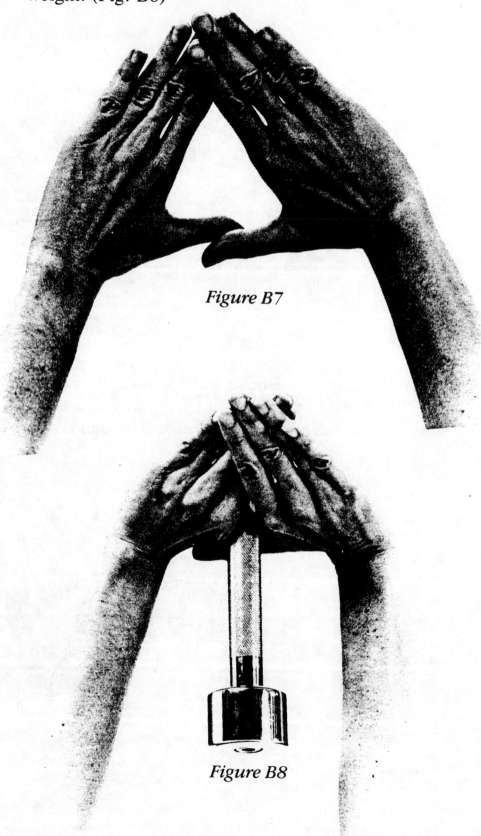

Figure B7

Figure B8

3. Begin with your arms straight above your chest. (Fig. B6)

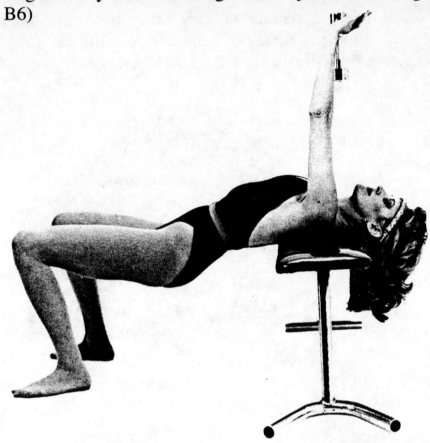

4. Keeping your elbows locked, lower the dumbbell backward and downward as far as you can move, then bend your elbows. (Figs. B9, B10, and B11)

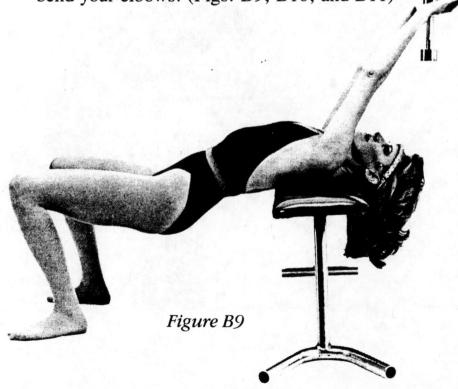

Figure B9

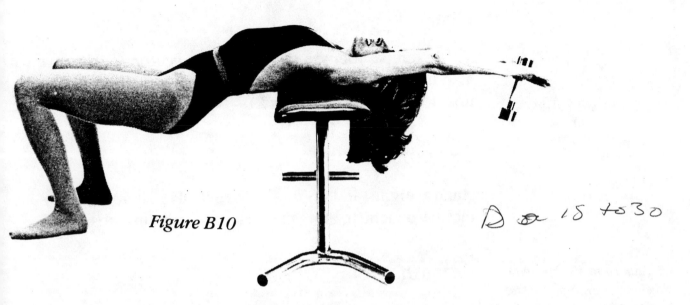

Figure B10

Do 15 to 30

5. Straighten your elbows and then return your arms so that they are straight above your chest.

Variation:

Perform the exercise the same as before, but lower your straight arms past your shoulders towards your legs for extra abdominal work.

then these

15 to 30

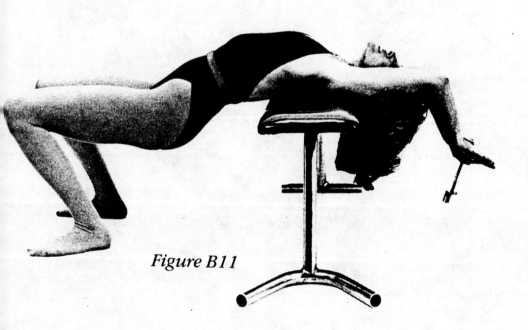

Figure B11

INCLINE FLYS

Goal:

This exercise focuses on your upper pectorals. However, it also uses your trapezius and teres major and minor (your upper bra line on your back).

Equipment:

Hand weights and an incline bench. If you do not have an incline bench, try this exercise in a standing position.

Amount:

10 to 12 reps; 1 to 2 sets

FLASH!
Of your 10 to 12 reps, do 4 slowly to warm up, 4 faster, but still smoothly, and 4 slowly for maximal emphasis!

30
10 slowly
10 faster
10 slowly

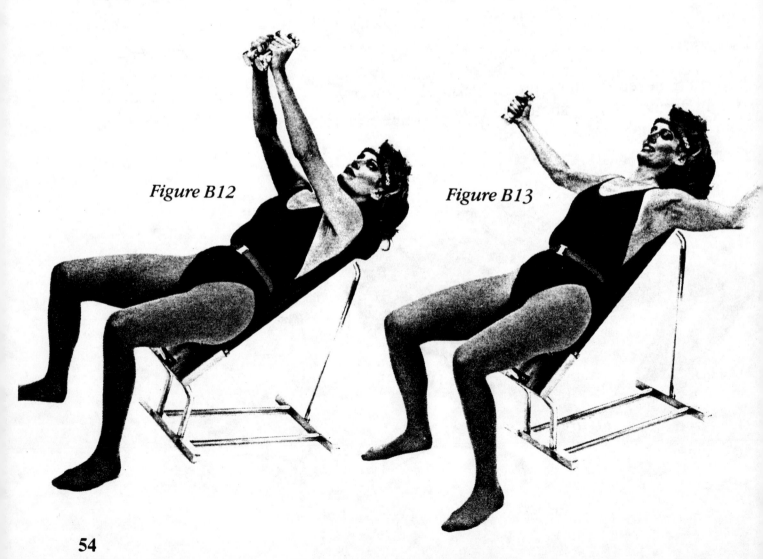

Figure B12   *Figure B13*

Instructions:

1. Rest on an incline bench. With a weight in each hand, your arms should be extended (remember to keep your elbows slightly bent throughout), and your palms should face each other in a parallel grip. (Fig. B12)
2. Simultaneously lower your hands to the sides of your shoulders and keep your elbows bent slightly. Lower your hands as far as possible to obtain the maximum benefit of this exercise. (Figs. B13 and B14)
3. Reversing the same movement, return your arms to above your shoulders.

bent elbows

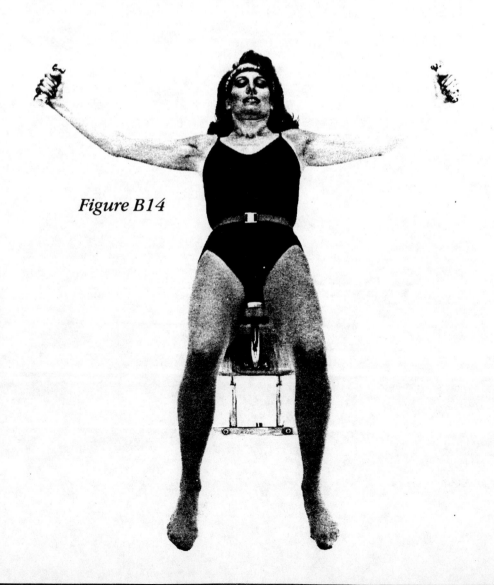

Figure B14

10
UPPER AND MIDDLE BACK

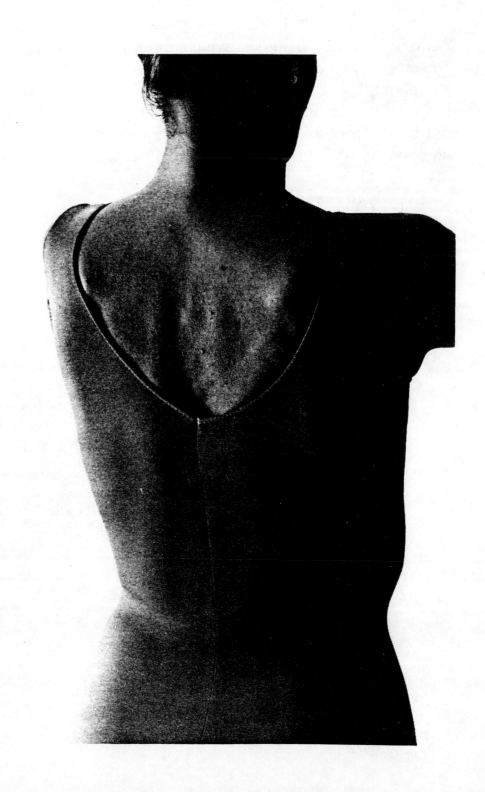

If you are like most women, you are aware of your back only when you're wearing a bathing suit or a strapless dress. Strong upper and middle back muscles are important, however, for your health. They enable you to lift relatively heavy objects without too much stress and strain on your back and to develop an upright, healthy, and attractive posture.

A strong back and shoulders which are developed in this set of exercises will enable you to stand and sit upright throughout the day without undue fatigue. Away with the stooped-shoulder image! Regular exercise also may prevent your bones from losing calcium and developing osteoporosis which is so prevalent in older women.

BENT-FORWARD DUMBBELL LATERAL RAISES

Goal:

To firm and develop the latissimus dorsi ("lats") which provide the pronounced V shape for your back that is noticeable in most body builders. You also will use your trapezius, deltoid, and erector spinae muscle groups, which add detail to the middle portion of your back.

Equipment:

Two small, 3-pound hand weights.

Amount:

10 to 12 reps; 1 to 2 sets

FLASH!
Push yourself as
hard as you can!

Instructions:

1. Start in a standing position and bend forward at your hips so that your upper body is parallel to the floor. (Figs. V1 and V2)

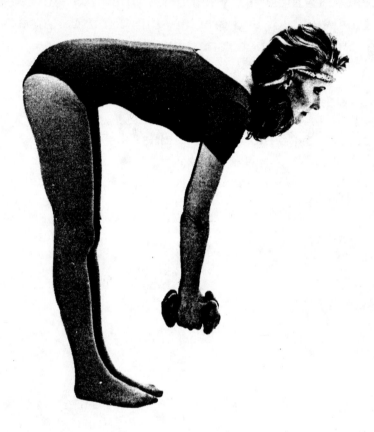

Figure V1

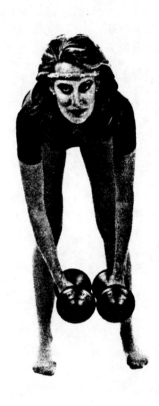

Figure V2

2.	Raise your arms to the sides of your shoulders. (Fig. V3)
3.	Remember to keep your elbows slightly bent as though you are carrying a big basket of laundry.

elbows bent

*faster on up
slower on down*

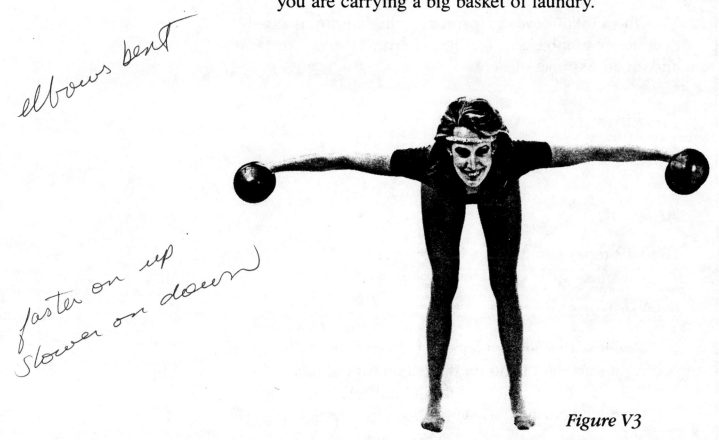

Figure V3

Tips:

- If you can do another rep after 10 or 12, don't stop.
- All movements should follow the "2–4" principle: If you take 2 seconds for the lifting portion of the movement, take 4 seconds for the lowering portion for maximum results.
- Your return to the starting position is more important than the lifting position of this exercise.

ONE-ARM BENT ROWING

Goal:

This movement develops primarily the latissimus dorsi. Secondary emphasis is on the forearm, biceps, trapezius, and erector spinae muscles.

Equipment:

5-pound weight and a flat bench or chair.

Amount:

10 to 12 reps; 1 to 2 sets with each arm.

Instructions:

1. Kneel with your head above the bench and place your right knee and hand on the bench for balance.
2. Put a 5- to 8-pound weight in your left hand, and start to move your hand down in front of your left leg. (Fig. V4)

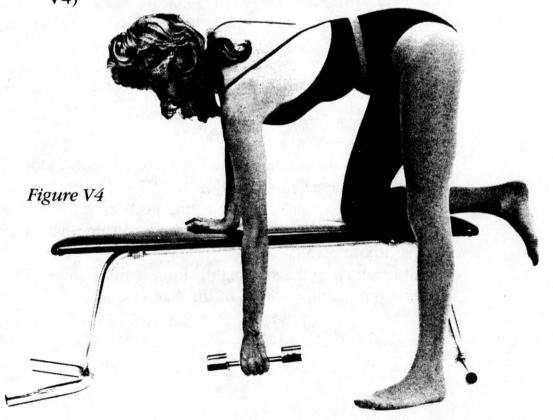

Figure V4

3. Slowly pick up the weight (Fig. V5) by bending your left arm and bringing your elbow up as high as you can. Your left hand is at bust level. This arm movement reminds me of pulling the power cord to start an electric lawn mower, only it is in slow motion.

Slowly

Contract abdominals & back

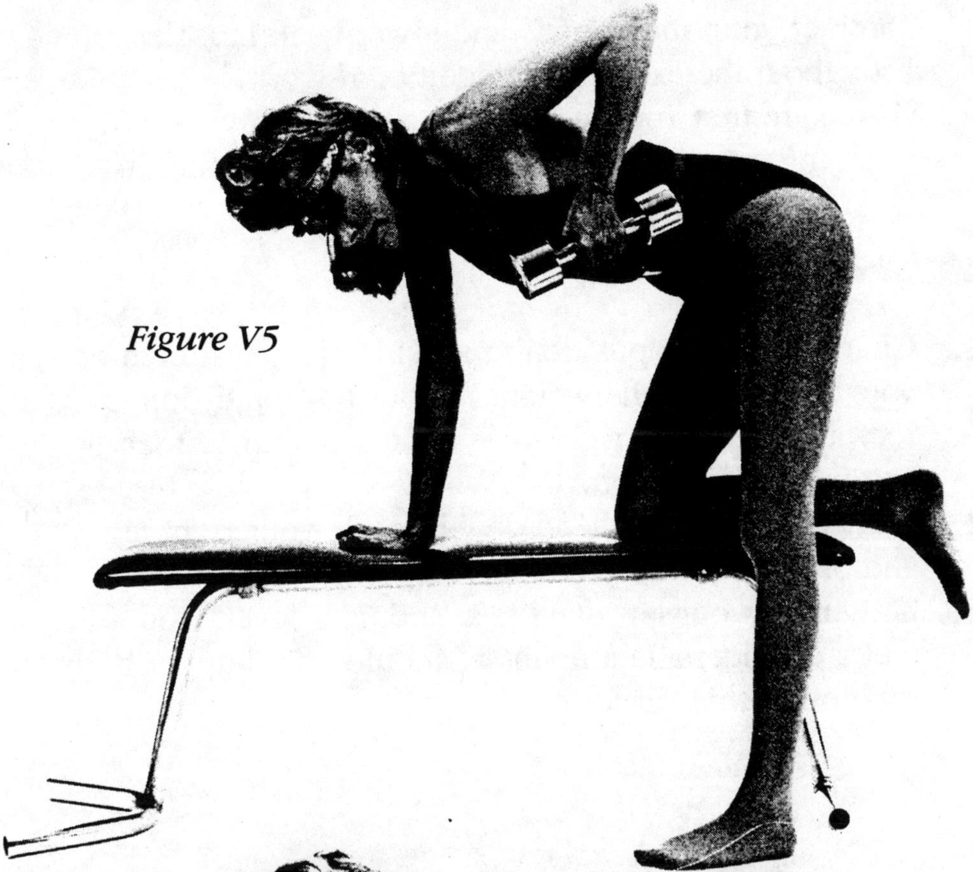

Figure V5

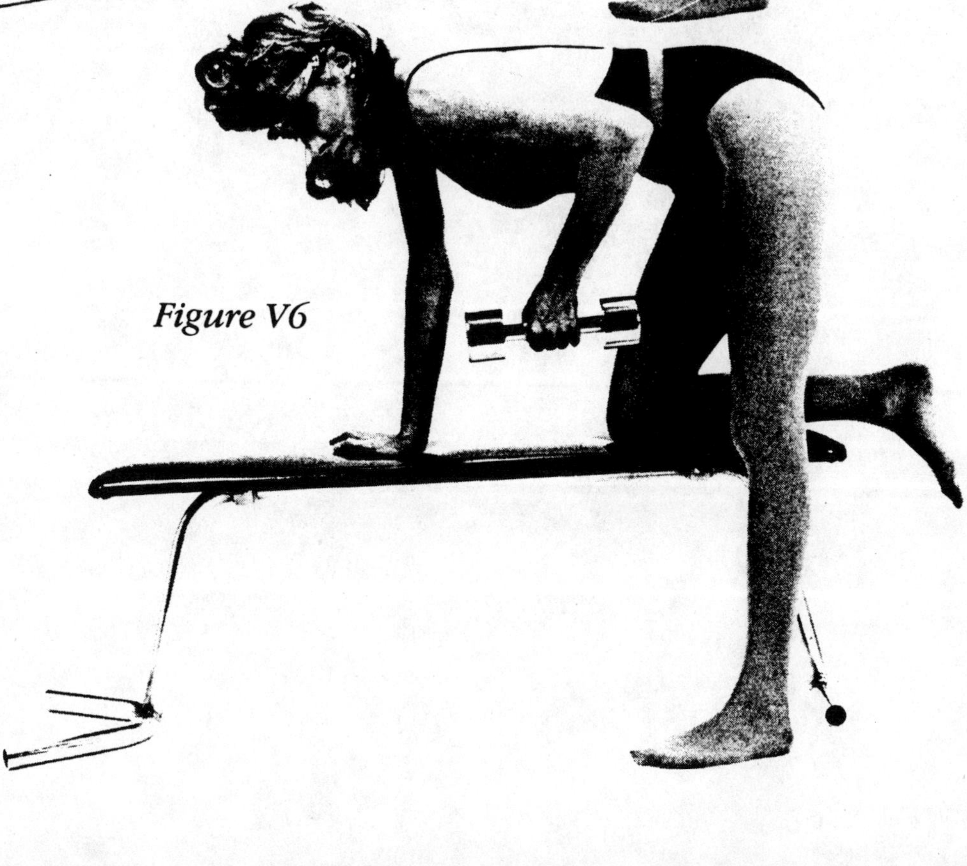

Figure V6

62

4. Lower the weight slowly to the starting position and repeat the movement. (Fig. V6)

Tips:

- Contract your abdominals and lower back muscles throughout the exercise for additional work.
- Make sure that your arm moves away from your body at a 45° angle to obtain maximum benefit for your lats.

Variation:

1. Change your leg position to include greater stretch on your back. With the weight in your left hand, lunge forward with your right knee bent and your left leg extended behind you.
2. Start with your left hand down beside your right leg and bring your left elbow up diagonally across your body until your left hand is at shoulder level. You will feel a considerable amount of shoulder and upper body rotation in this variation.

SEATED BENT LATERALS

Goal:

This exercise is great for your posterior deltoids and your entire upper back.

Amount:

10 to 12 reps; 1 to 2 sets

Equipment:

Flat bench and *light* (3-pound) hand weights.

FLASH!
Weights should be heavy, but not too heavy for good form!

Instructions:

1. Sit at the end of a flat bench with your feet and legs together. Lean forward until your torso rests on your thighs. Touch the two dumbbells together behind your ankles. (Fig. V7)
2. Raise your arms directly to the side in a semicircle until your arms are at shoulder height (remember to keep your elbows slightly bent). (Fig. V8)
3. Lower your arms to the starting position and repeat.

Tips:

*   When you are raising your arms, keep them 90° to your torso, or slightly toward your head rather than your hips.
*   This exercise can be done sitting on the edge of an armless chair.

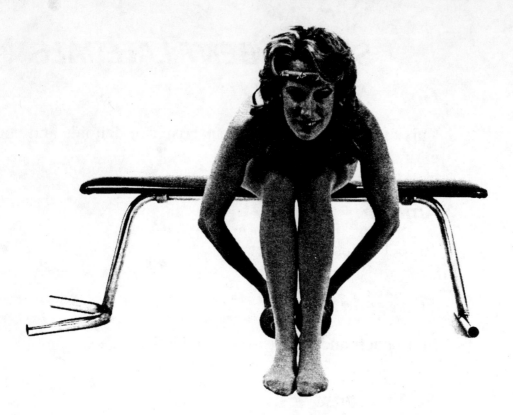

Figure V7

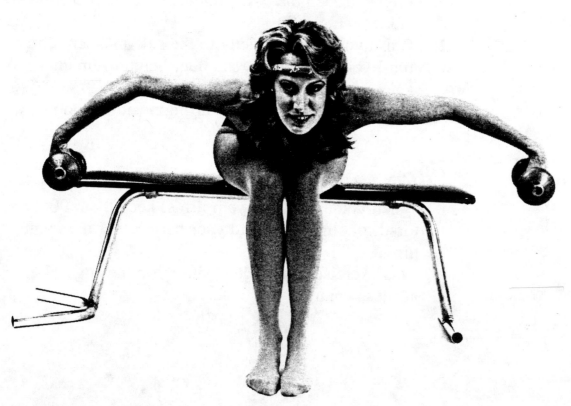

Figure V8

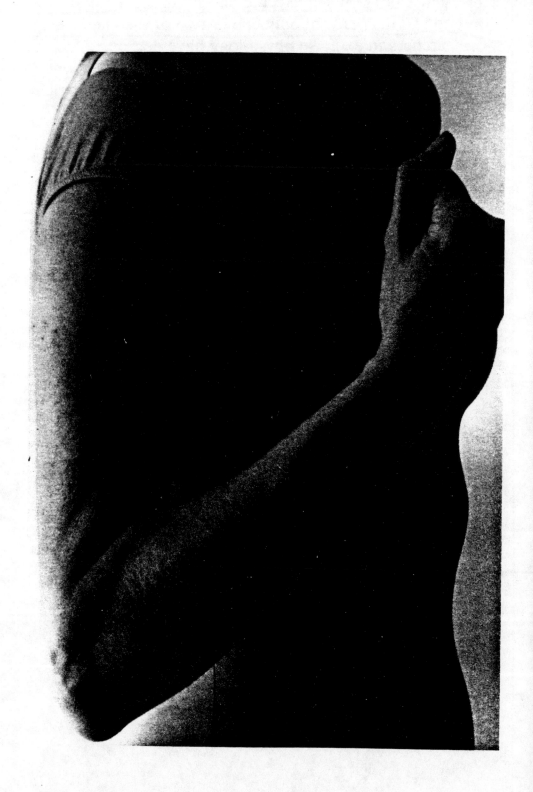

Flabby upper arms are a problem area for many women, and are ~~difficult~~ to firm. If you suffer from flabby arms, be sure to complete two sets of each exercise. The sooner you start, the sooner you will see progress.

Initially you may find it difficult to complete even one set of each. Until you can execute one set of all three exercises in good form, perform only one or two of the exercises. Researchers in exercise physiology have demonstrated that women are weak in the upper arm and shoulder region. Since our lack of strength is more cultural than biological, it is easily remedied.

If your upper arms are in fantastic shape, I recommend a set or two of the CONCENTRATION CURL and the TRICEPS EXTENSION to keep them that way. Of course, you may decide to do all three.

CONCENTRATION CURL

Goal:

This exercise focuses specifically on your biceps and triceps as you flex and extend your elbow.

Equipment:

Medium (approximately 5-pound) hand weights.

Amount:

10 to 12 reps; 1 to 2 sets with each arm

FLASH!
If one arm is weaker
than the other,
exercise the
weaker one first!

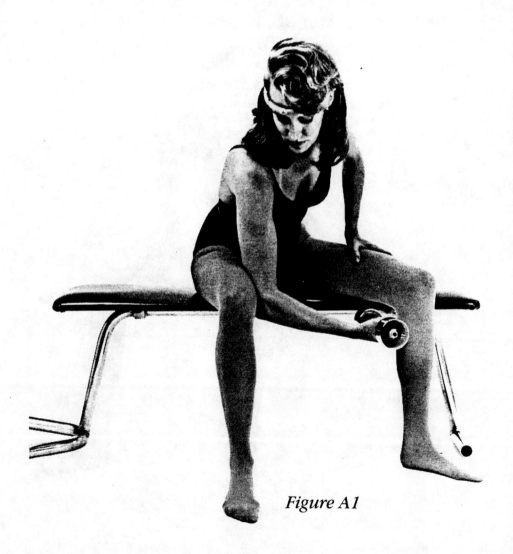

Figure A1

Instructions:

1. To begin, sit on the side of your bench. Rest the elbow of the arm holding the weight against the inside of your thigh, midway between the top and bottom. This helps you keep your upper arm immobile. Your elbow is about four inches above your knee. (Fig. A1)
2. Keeping your elbow against your thigh, slowly lower your arm to your ankle. (Fig. A2)

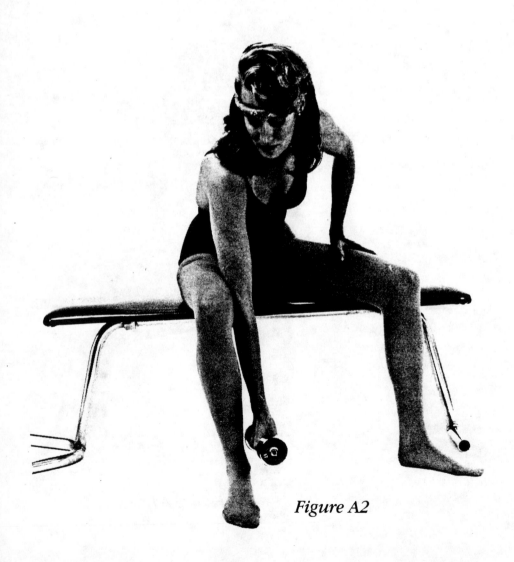

Figure A2

3. Complete the exercise by raising the weight to your chest. (Figs. A3 and A4)

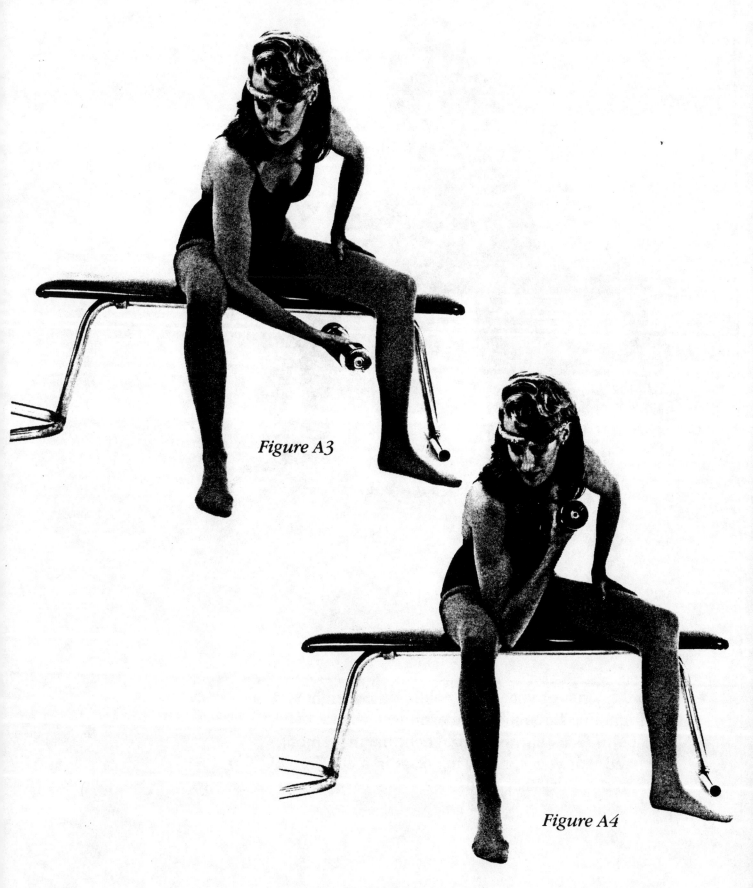

Figure A3

Figure A4

4. Return to the starting position. (Fig. A5).

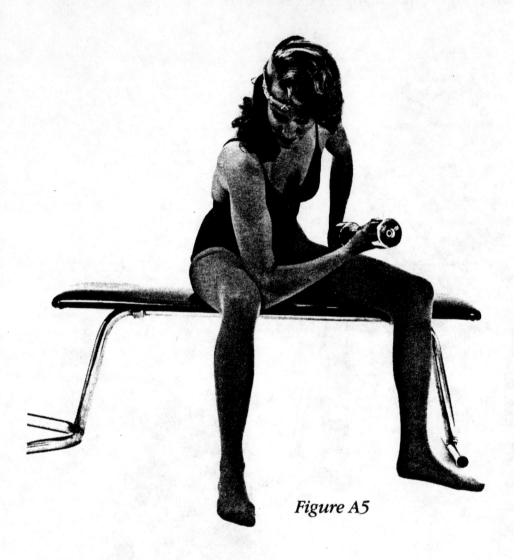

Figure A5

Tips:

- Keep the wrist of your hand holding the weight straight and immobile throughout the exercise.
- Your palm faces upward throughout the movement.
- The hand that you're not using rests in a comfortable position on your other thigh.

STANDING ALTERNATE DUMBBELL CURL

Goal:

To tone your biceps and, secondarily, your triceps.

Equipment:

Two 5- to 8-pound hand weights.

Amount:

20 to 24 reps alternating arms; 1 to 2 sets

FLASH!
Be brave and work out
in a bathing suit;
see your muscles work!

Instructions:

1. Start with both hands, each holding a weight, at the sides of your body (i.e., beside your thighs). The palms of your hands face forward. (Fig. A6)
2. Using one arm at a time, keep your thumb up as you bend your elbow, bringing your hand to your shoulder. (Figs. A7 and A8)
3. Return arm to side of body and alternate your arms using an exceedingly slow, seesaw type of movement.

Tips:

- Keep your elbows in close to your body.
- Do not bend your wrist.
- Contract your abdominals throughout for additional benefits.

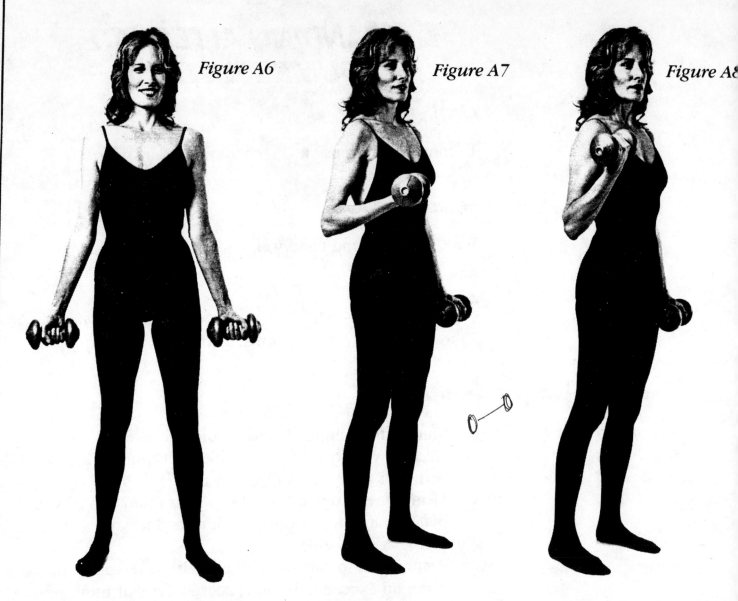

Figure A6   Figure A7   Figure A8

Variation: Hammer Curl

This alternate version emphasizes the outside of your upper arm and your forearm more than does the regular standing alternate dumbbell curl. It can be done in addition to or instead of the standing dumbbell curl for a little variety. Start with your arms at your sides and your thumbs facing forward. As you bring your lower arm up, rotate your wrist outward so that your palms are facing up.

Slow
Contract
abdominals

Do these also
start and

73

TRICEPS EXTENSION

Goal:

To firm your triceps, with a secondary focus on your pectoral and deltoid muscles.

Equipment:

Start with a 3- or 5-pound free weight.

Amount:

10 to 12 reps; 1 to 2 sets

Instructions:

1. Begin in a standing position, feet should be shoulder distance apart. Hold a weight in one hand and raise it straight above your head. (Fig. A9)
2. Clasp the triceps of your arm holding the weight with your free hand to keep your extended arm close to your head and absolutely stationary. (Fig. A10)

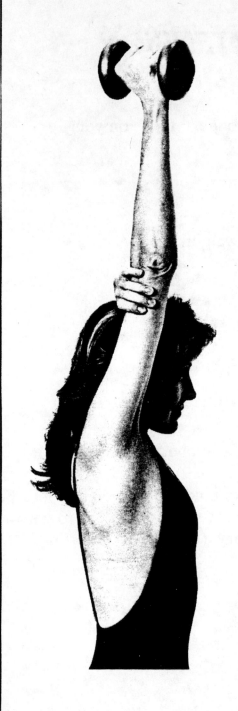

Figure A9

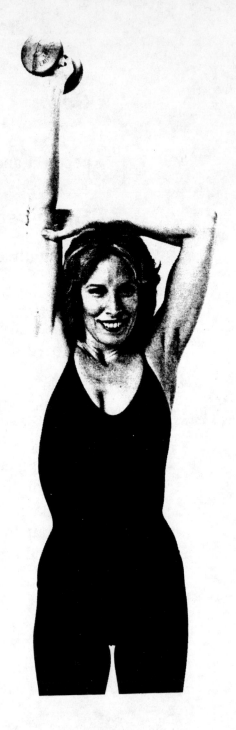

Figure A10

3. Slowly lower the dumbbell toward your shoulder and then raise it again. (Figs. A11 and A12)

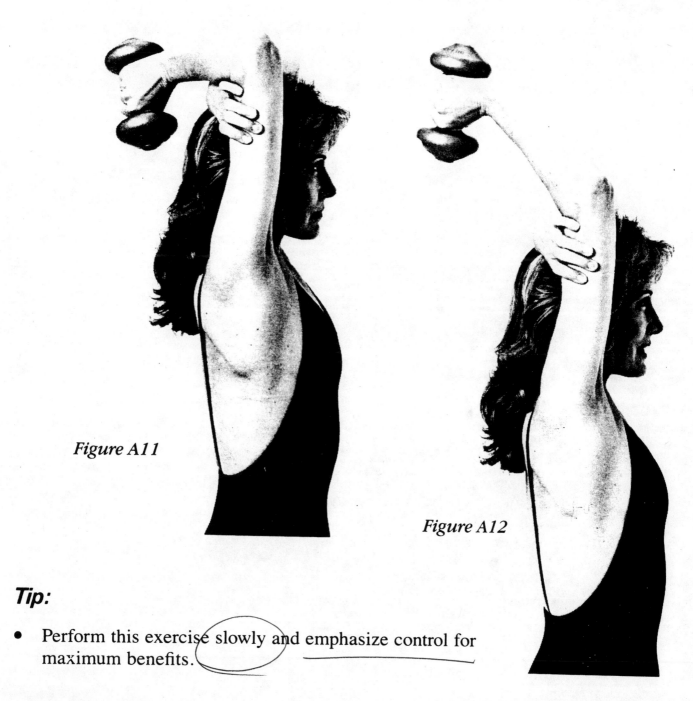

Figure A11

Figure A12

Tip:

- Perform this exercise slowly and emphasize control for maximum benefits.

Variation:

Hold a weight in each hand and extend arms upward simultaneously. Be sure to keep your upper arms stationary. However, you may find that you work your triceps harder when you concentrate on one arm at a time as in the regular triceps extension.

12
WAIST

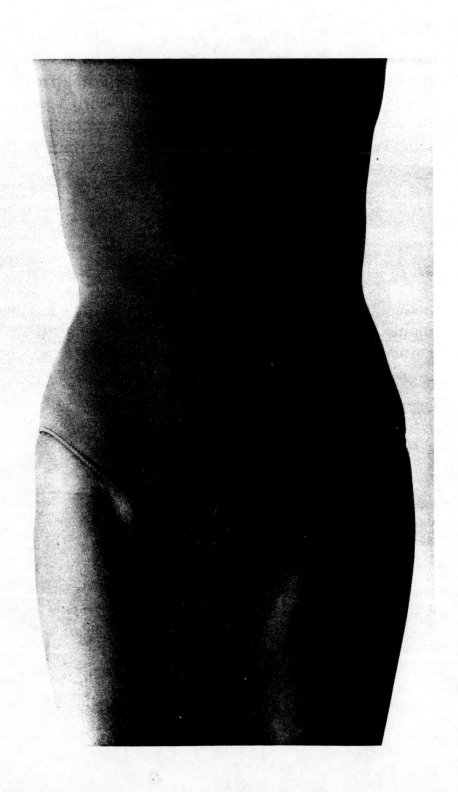

This section will help indent the *side* portion of your waist since the front panel is controlled by your abdominal muscles. Your external oblique muscles run along the side of your body here, and strengthening them increases the amount of indentation at the side of your waist. I've been doing these two exercises for years and believe in them. They work!

Exercises for this portion of your body will firm your muscles, but they will not eliminate globs of fat. To get rid of excess flesh, you need to DIET. Exercise primarily firms what muscles you have. Of course, you will burn a few more calories than you usually do while you exercise, but reducing your caloric intake is important if you want to achieve a noticeable weight loss.

SIDE LEANS

Goal:

To strengthen your external oblique muscle group, and thus to emphasize the amount of indentation at the sides of your waist.

FLASH!
Set realistic goals
for yourself.
Aim to look your best!

Equipment:

Two 3- to 5-pound hand weights.

Amount:

10 to 12 reps; 2 to 3 sets

Instructions:

1. Starting position: Stand with your feet shoulder distance apart, left hand on waist. (Fig. W1)
2. Hold the weight in your right hand with your arm extended above your head. Your right elbow is slightly bent.
3. The less you bend your elbow, the more difficult the movement. Experiment to see what's best for you.
4. With your left hand on your waist lean to the left as far as you can go easily. (Figs. W2 and W3) (The hand on your waist is for balance, not support.)
5. Return to the center and repeat ten times before switching sides.

Speed matters not how fast you bend

fast

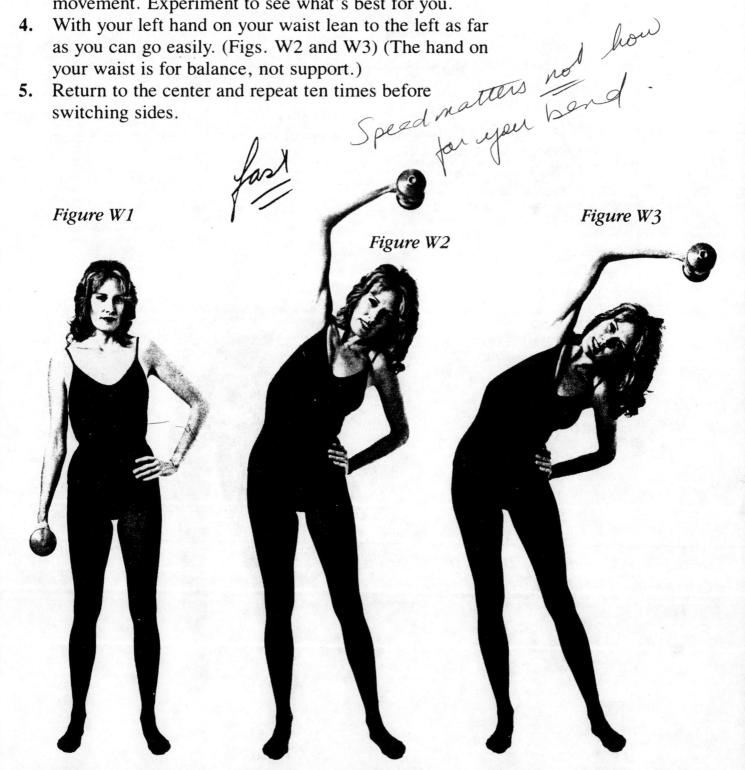

Figure W1

Figure W2

Figure W3

Hints:

- This is one of the few exercises in which your movements should be rapid. Moving vigorously to the side and back again is far more important than how far to the side you go.
- Practice this without a weight if you experience any difficulties.

Variation:

Starting position is the same as for Side Leans (Fig. W1). Lean toward the side with the weight, letting the weight drop as low as possible. Remember to keep your shoulders facing forward. Repeat this rapidly, ten times, before changing sides. (Fig. W4)

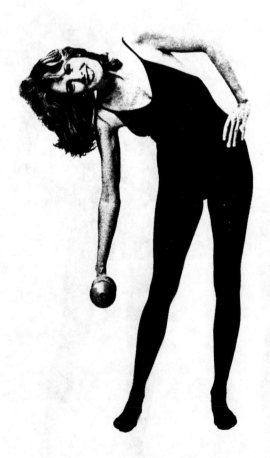

Figure W4

80

LATERAL TURNS

Goal:

The primary emphasis is on your external obliques.
However, your erector spinae are also working to effect
torso rotation. The secondary emphasis of this movement is
on your abdominal and lower-back muscles.

Equipment:

Heavier hand weights of approximately 8 to 10 pounds.

Amount:

10 to 15 reps; 2 to 4 sets

FLASH!
Work out three days
a week with a
day of rest in between!

Instructions:

1. Hold a dumbbell in each hand at shoulder height. (Fig. W5)
2. Turn your upper body slowly as far as you can to one side and then to the other side. (Fig W6)
3. Use your hip and thigh muscles to hold your lower body motionless. This is crucial to performing the exercise properly.
4. Count moving to the left *and* right as a single repetition.

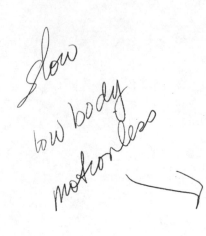

slow
low body
motionless

Hints:

1. Pinch your buttocks together and you will reap additional benefits.
2. Do not allow your hips to turn.

Variation:

Try holding the weights beside your thighs, swing to left and then to right, and you will use slightly different muscles.

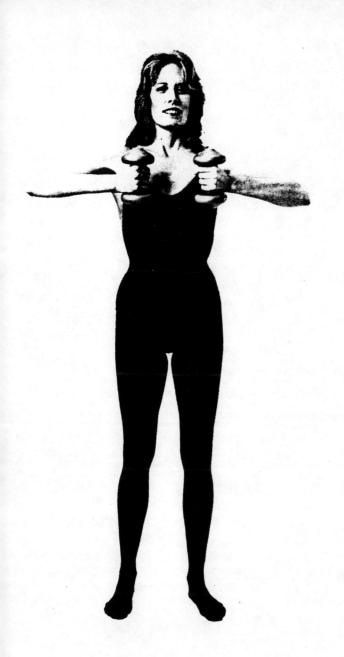

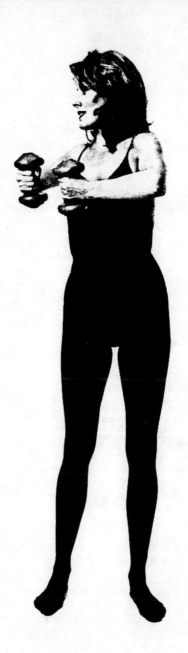

Figure W5

Figure W6

13
HIPS, HIPS, HURRAY!

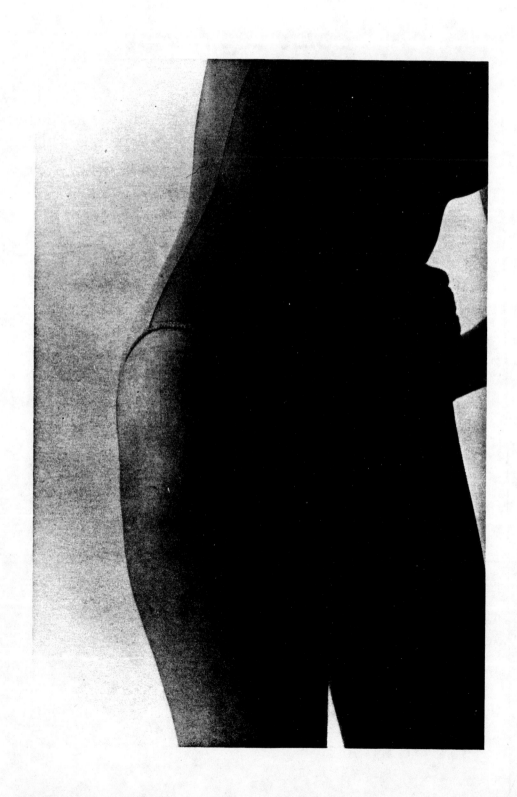

This set of exercises focuses on the outer portion of your body between your waist and thighs. Although your general body build determines the exact size of your hips, you can do wonders by keeping them firm and trim. Dancers, swimmers, and gymnasts use their hips in their individual activities and have gorgeous hips. The next two exercises will help you do a super job of toning your hips.

Side Leg Raises

Goal:

Toning the gluteal group, especially the gluteus medius which abducts the thigh and the gluteus maximus which extends your hip. Your hamstrings are a secondary group of muscles that you will firm.

Equipment:

2-pound ankle weights or a pair of heavy shoes. When you're ready, use 4-pound ankle weights.

Amount:

20 reps; 2 to 3 sets

FLASH!
Soaking in a hot bath will alleviate muscle soreness!

Instructions:

1. Lie on your side with your body in a perfectly straight line from head to toe. Be sure that your buttocks are not sticking out. Support the upper portion of your body on your bottom elbow by placing your hand against your ear to support your head. Place your other hand on the floor in front of you for support. (Fig. H1)
2. Slowly raise your top leg as high as you can. (Fig. H2)
3. Lower your leg to the floor, but avoid touching it to the floor before repeating the movement.

Tips:

Up – med speed
down – slow

- Since the downward movement is more important than the upward one, perform this movement even more slowly.
- The higher you raise your top leg, the higher on your hips the muscles will be working.
    a. If you can raise your top leg to the perpendicular, you will extend the benefits to your waist.
- Increase the amount of ankle weight as you progress.

Variation:

Extend your top arm upward away from your hip and try to touch your leg to it. (Fig. H3)

Figure H1

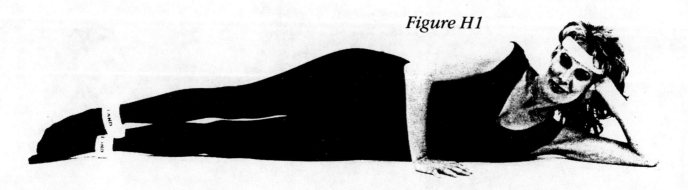

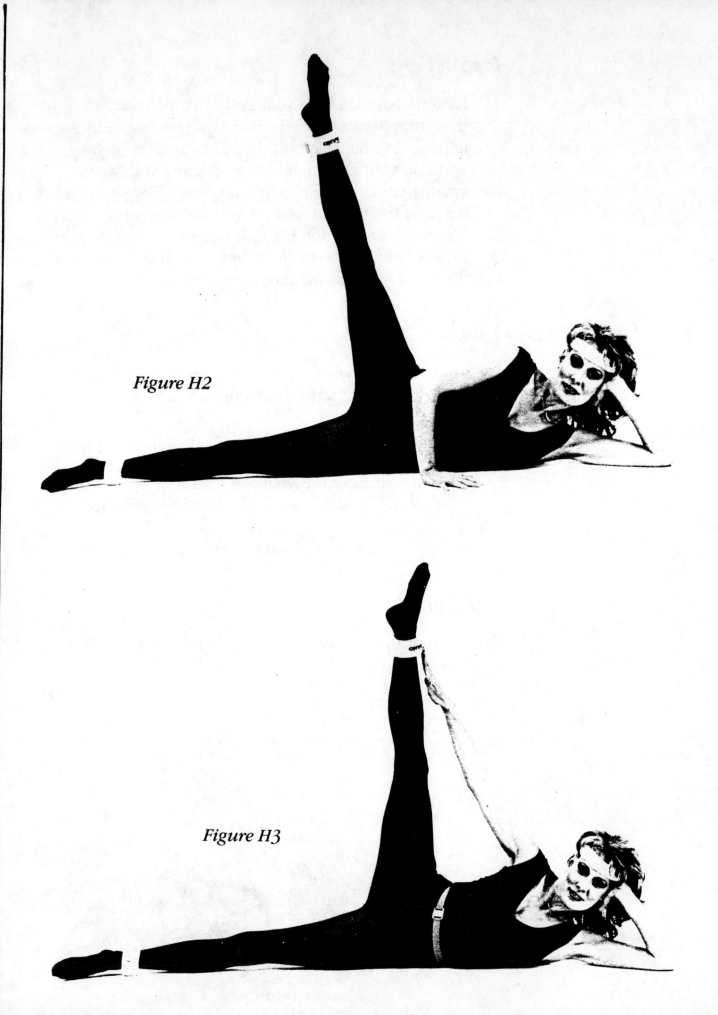

Figure H2

Figure H3

Tuck Side Leg Raises

This exercise is very similar to the previous one. However, in addition to toning your gluteus medius, it focuses more strongly on your gluteus maximus, hamstrings, and quadriceps. This exercise is a real toughie!

Equipment:

2-pound ankle weights.

Amount:

15 to 20 reps; 1 to 4 sets

FLASH!
Think of how gorgeous
you will look!

Instructions:

1. Lie on your side with your body in a perfectly straight line from head to toe. Support the upper portion of your body by resting your head on your hand. (Fig. H4)
2. Begin by raising your knee to your chin. (Fig. H5)
3. Lower it to your foot. (Fig. H6)

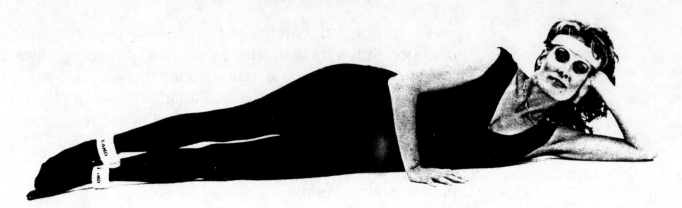

Figure H4

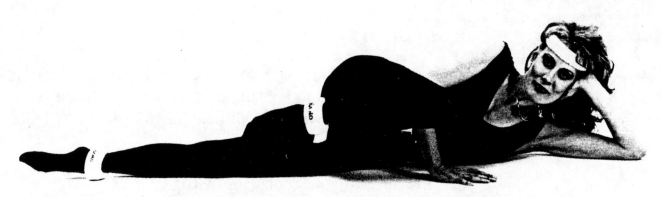

Figure H5

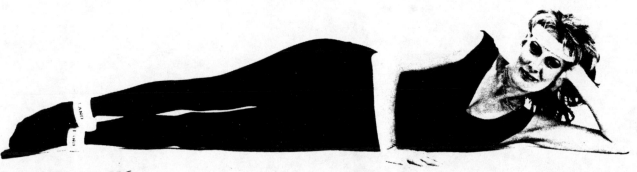

Figure H6

4. Raise your extended leg upward from your hip. (Fig. H7)
5. Lower your leg to the floor and repeat the same movement before turning onto your other side.

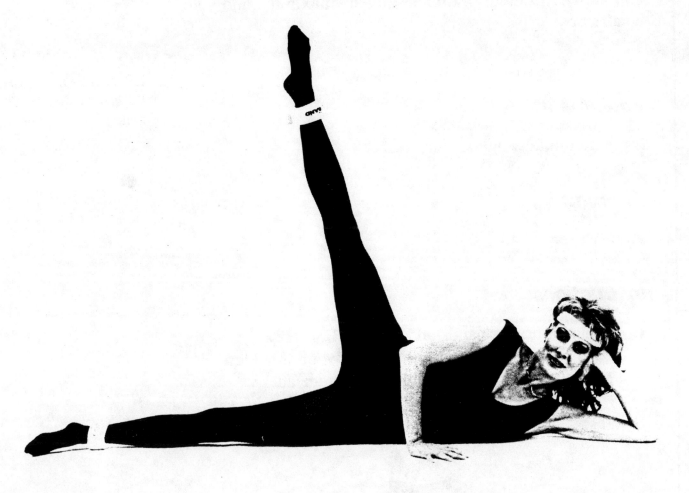

Figure H7

Fire Hydrant

Goal:

To tone your gluteus minimus, gluteus maximus, and your quadriceps.

FLASH!
The heavier the weight, the greater the toning!

Equipment:

2-pound ankle weights.

Amount:

10 to 15 reps; 1 to 2 sets

Instructions:

1. Crouch on your hands and knees. (Fig. H8)
    - Your arms are perpendicular to your shoulders.
    - Your fingers are pointing straight ahead.
    - Your thighs are perpendicular to your body.

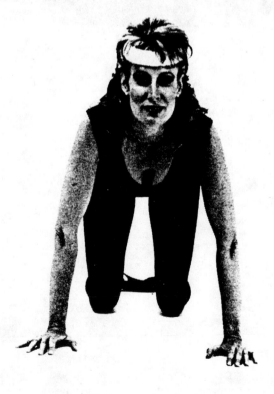

Figure H8

3. Slowly, and with great control, lower it to the floor and repeat this motion for an entire set of forward leg raises. In addition to focusing on your quadriceps, this portion focuses on your abdominals, especially if you contract them throughout your movement. (Fig. T3)

up

slow down

contract abdominals

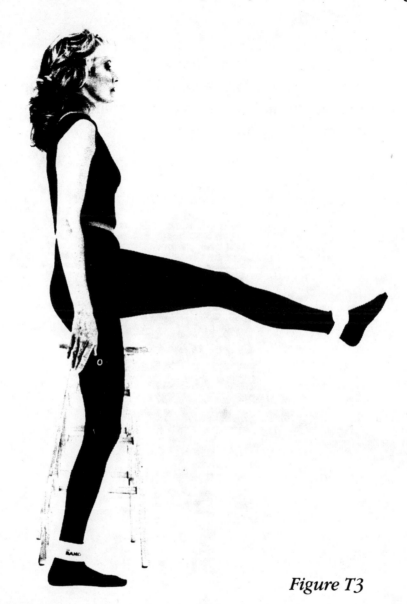

Figure T3

4. Complete another set of leg raises to the side to firm your inner and outer thigh. In addition to your adductor magnus and quadriceps, this movement includes hip and waist muscles if you keep your upper body motionless. (Fig. T4)

5. Complete a third set of leg raises to the rear for hamstring emphasis before repeating the sequence with your other leg. This portion also uses your buttocks. (Fig. T5)

Tips:

- Originate all leg movement from your hip. If you truly hold your lower body motionless, you should feel strong muscle contractions in the hip of your stationary leg.
- Contract your abdominals for double duty.

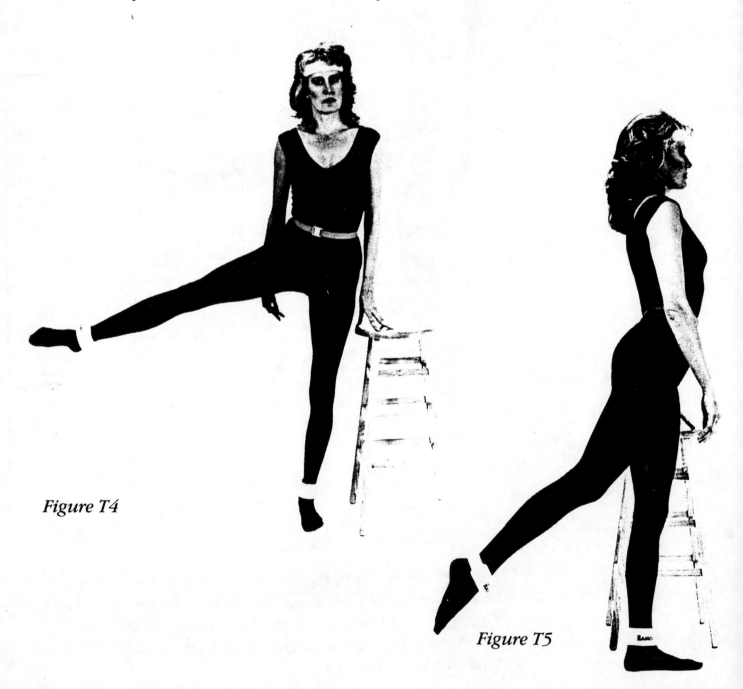

Figure T4

Figure T5

LUNGE

Goal:

You will really feel your thigh muscles working in this movement. This exercise defines your quadriceps—particularly near your hip. It also firms and rounds your buttocks.

Equipment:

Although the Lunge is most often done with a barbell behind your neck, it also can be done at home with a pair of dumbbells in your hands. Initially try this exercise using 5- to 8-pound weights. You will progress to 10- to 15-pound weights soon.

FLASH!
Keep a mental image
of the thighs
you want to develop!

Amount:

10 to 12 reps; 1 to 2 sets

Instructions:

1. Stand with your feet shoulder distance apart. Hold the weights in each hand at the sides of your thighs. (Fig. T6)
2. Step forward as far as possible with your right foot. Bend your right knee so that it is several inches ahead of your foot. Don't allow your knee to bend so much that your thigh is less than parallel to the floor. Protect your knee by *never* doing a full knee bend. (Fig. T7)
3. Keep your right leg as straight as possible.
4. Push back to the starting point.
5. Repeat with the alternate leg.

Tips:

• If you feel strain on your lower back, lean forward a little with your torso.

- Feel the stretch along the entire back of your extended leg. The closer you keep the heel of your back leg on the floor, the more you will be toning your calf muscle.
- To increase the difficulty of the Lunge, hold heavier weights, or maintain the bent-knee position for three to five seconds before you return to the starting position.

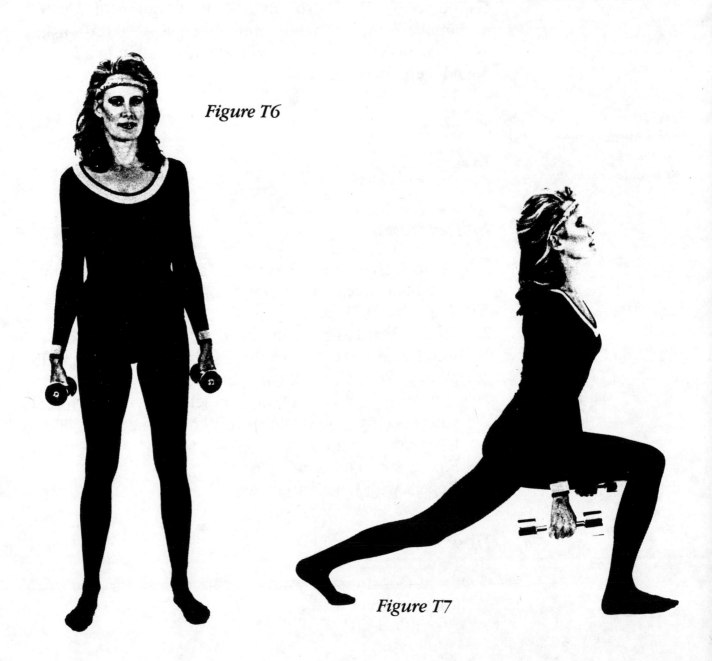

Figure T6

Figure T7

16
LOWER LEG

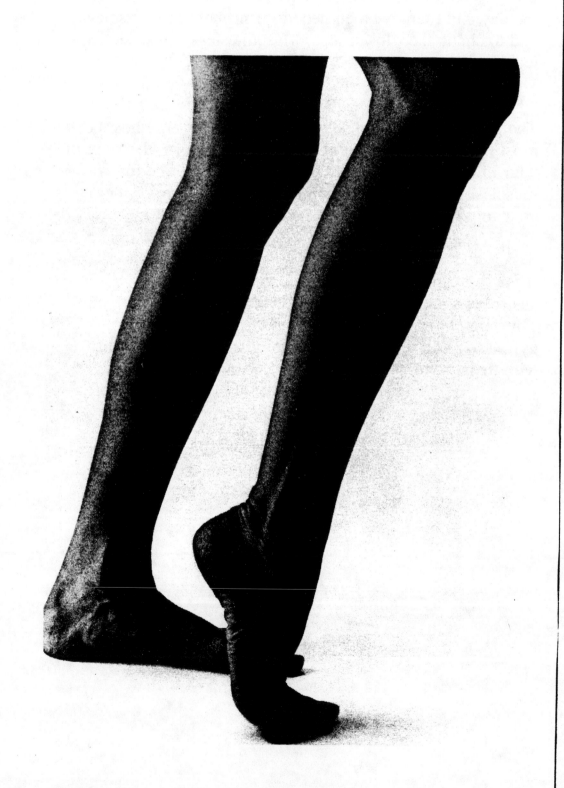

Anytime you wear a skirt, your lower legs are highly visible! Like most of your body, either you were born with good legs, or you weren't.

You can firm and lengthen the muscles that you have even though you cannot change your bone structure. You are likely to exercise your lower legs as you walk throughout the day, but many women need to firm their calf muscles and to shape their lower legs. Muscular legs are attractive legs!

The gastrocnemius and soleus are the largest and thus the most important of the eight muscles which form the back of your lower leg. Both act to extend your foot. The four front muscles, the largest of which is the tibialis anterior, flex your foot (i.e., bring your toes toward your body).

If you wear high heels, you need to stretch your gastrocnemius and soleus to prevent them from shortening. This stretching is particularly important for joggers, gymnasts, and tennis players who wish to prevent problems with their Achilles tendon.

ONE-LEG CALF RAISE

Goal:

General toning, stretching, and development of your calves.

Equipment:

Ankle weights and a block of wood or a large, thick book. This exercise can be performed standing backward on the edge of a step if there is a handrail to use for balance.

Amount:

10 to 12 reps; 1 to 2 sets

Instructions:

1. Hold onto something for balance. (A dining-room chair is fine.) Place the forward portion of the foot you are exercising on a thick piece of wood or large book. Your toes are pointing straight ahead. Bend the knee of your other leg to raise it out of the way. (Fig. L1)

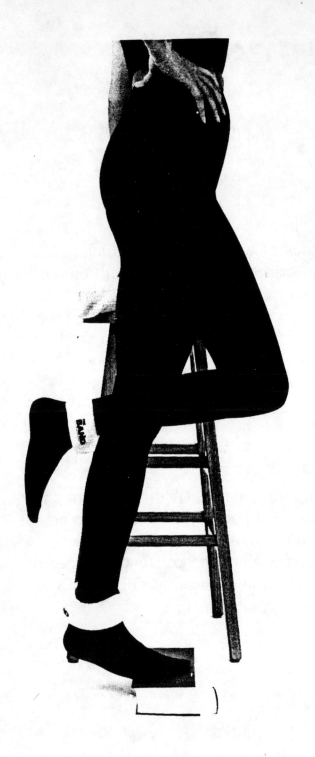

FLASH!
Lower your heel as far as you can to counterbalance the effects of high heels!

Figure L1

2. Stand up on your toes as high as you can. Feel the "burn." (Fig. L2)

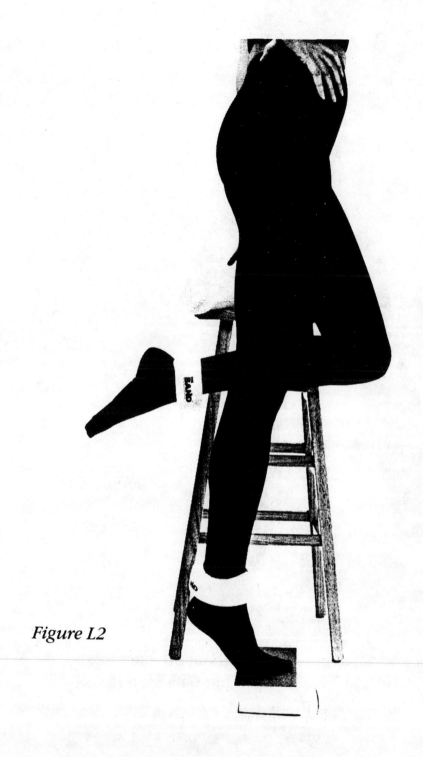

Figure L2

3. Then, lower your heel as far below your toes as possible. Really stretch! This is the portion of the movement which helps to prevent Achilles-tendon problems. If your heels touch the floor, you need a thicker piece of wood or book. (Fig. L3)

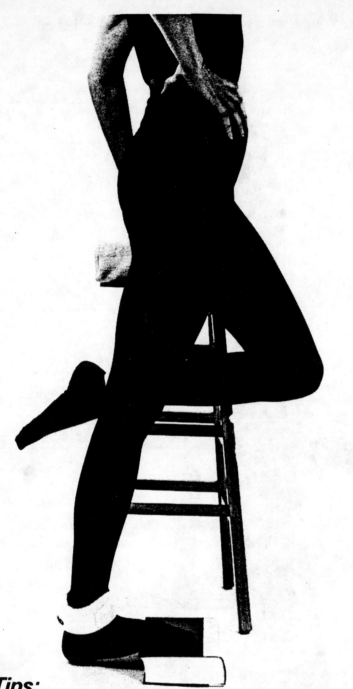

Figure L3

Tips:

- Contract your abdominals throughout all exercises.
- This exercise can be done standing on a step if you have a handrail for support.

Variations:

1. Turn your foot 45° to the outside and repeat the movement. It's easier to balance if you perform this exercise on two feet.
2. Turn your foot 45° to the inside.

ANKLE CIRCLES

Goal:

To develop trim, firm ankles.

Equipment:

2- to 4-pound ankle weights.

Amount:

10 to 12 reps; 1 to 2 sets

Instructions:

1. Sit on a chair and cross your right leg over the left. Rotate the foot of your top leg clockwise. Point your toes down, toward the inside of your ankle, up, and toward the outside of your ankle. (Figs. L4, L5, and L6)
2. Perform this movement very slowly and feel all the muscles in your calf and ankle.
3. Reverse the direction of the circle in the second set before switching legs.

Tip:

- If you are prone to spraining your ankle, avoid the circles in which you move your foot to the bottom, outside of your leg, and then upward.

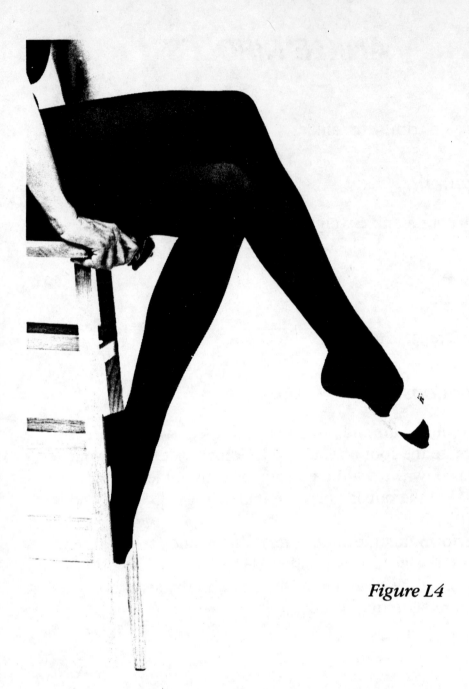

Figure L4

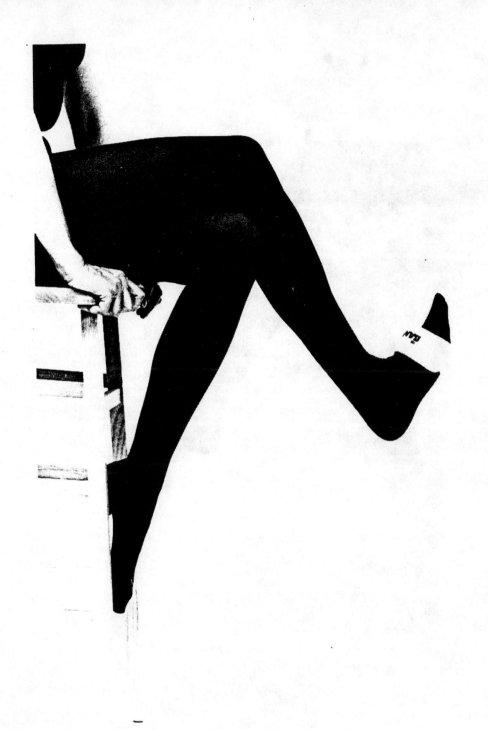

Figure L5

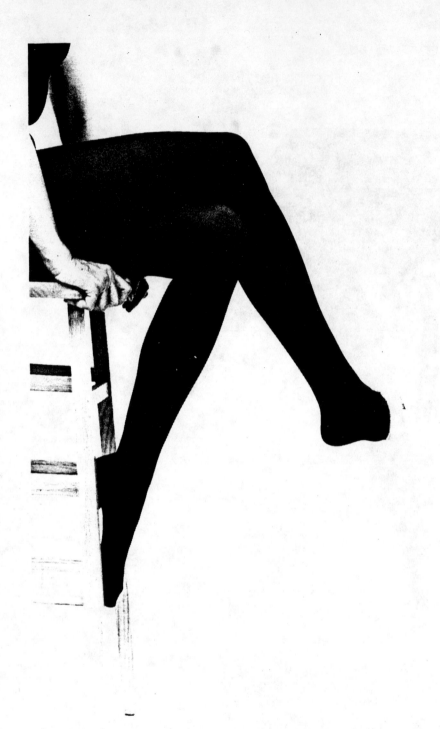

Figure L6

Part III
The New You

17
A Little Bit About Posing Like the Body Builders

Body builders consider posing a competitive sport, a form of self-expression, and an art form. They are creating and sculpting their own bodies. Rather than leave their work at home, as do most artists, they have the privilege of carrying their bodies with them wherever they go. Regardless of whether you are thinking seriously of becoming a competitive body builder, it is important to know a little about the sport in order to know how to proceed should you ever become more interested.

Women officially began competing in the sport of body-building in 1978, and since that time the rules about posing have evolved. Initially there was considerable confusion as to whether women's standards for judging should be the same as for men.

If you decide to compete, you will find that the imposed time schedule is a wonderful motivator. You train harder than before, and the competition is fun. You will also begin to give more serious attention to your diet in order to reduce your overall body fat and to emphasize muscle definition. Even if you have no plans to ever enter competition, just knowing about judging standards and procedures will help you to personalize your own workout.

Throughout the three rounds of competition, body builders are judged according to (1) the symmetry of their muscles (i.e., left and right sides should be similar); (2) body proportion (both upper and lower body parts should be equally developed); (3) maximum muscular development; and, of course, (4) hard muscles. In varying degrees, these are the things that we all would like!

In Round I, the contestants are rated by a panel of judges while they stand in a relaxed position. (In Rounds I and II, the competitors are judged individually and in small groups for comparison purposes. Round III is completely individual.) The judges consider such things as body symmetry, proportional balance, and general muscle tone. The winners of Round I advance to the next round.

In Round II, the body builders perform a series of compulsory poses in order that the competitors may be judged according to equal conditions. The artistic aspect of this round lies in interpreting the compulsory poses in such a way that each woman's assets are displayed to their best advantage. You can write to the American Federation of Women Bodybuilders, Box 937, Riverview, Florida 33569 for a Judging Guide which lists the current compulsory poses.

In Round III, each woman free-poses to music of her choice. Each of the three rounds count one third of her total bodybuilding score.

For additional information, refer to Laura Combes's book, *Winning Women's Bodybuilding*, which is listed in the Suggested Readings. Laura has won numerous bodybuilding titles, including Ms. America, and shares her training enthusiasm and tips. Other excellent sources of information are *Muscle and Fitness* magazine and *Nautilus* magazine.

Many competitive body builders train six to eight hours a day to develop their muscles, to experiment with various poses, and to fit their poses to music. A particularly difficult aspect of posing is to be able to flex each muscle while keeping your face relaxed. Most body builders acquire a fairly dark tan to show their muscles to better advantage. Of course, body makeup does the same thing and is much kinder to your skin. If you think that you may be seriously interested in competing, be sure to attend a competitive event to acquire additional information.

18
Feeling Good About Yourself Will Help You Look Better

After you have been weight training for four or five weeks, you will notice a host of differences—physical, psychological, and behavioral. Your muscles will be firmer and more shapely, you will get rid of flab, your posture will improve automatically, and you will notice a new store of energy. Weight training does wonders for your self-concept and body awareness. In short, you will look and feel great.

The relationship between looking and feeling better from weight training is circular. One complements the other, and it is hard to tell exactly which occurs first. Feeling better helps you look even better.

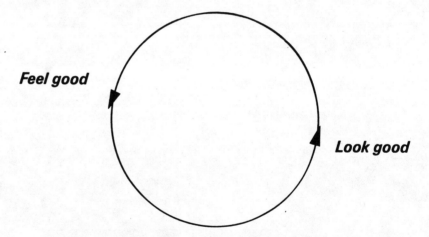

Feel good

Look good

The Weight-Training Cycle

Think about the days on which you have felt great in the past. The chances are that you have had a more positive attitude than usual, felt energetic, were pleased with yourself, and accomplished more than usual. Friends may have commented on how good you looked! You might have thought that you got out on the right side of the bed, that your biorhythms were aligned with one another, or that there was considerable truth in the "power of positive thinking." Regardless of the underlying dynamics, you undoubtedly feel, look, and perform better on some days than others.

Your weight-lifting program enables you to create more "good" days for yourself. As you stick with the program, you'll be pleased with your dedication and will note a true feeling of accomplishment as you take charge of your body and your life. By regularly scheduling a weight-training session into your busy day, you are indicating to yourself that you value yourself, you're taking care of your health, and not allowing something important to be pushed aside by the myriad of things that you MUST do. Weight training definitely enhances your physical and psychological well-being.

You may not become a competitive body builder, but you can experience the joys!

Suggested Readings

Berger, Bonnie G. "Facts and Fancy: Mood Alteration through Exercise." In *Journal of Physical Education, Recreation, and Dance* 53: 47–48, November–December, 1982.

— . "Running Away from Anxiety and Depression: A Female as Well as Male Race." In *Running Therapy and Psychology,* eds. M. Sachs and G. Buffone. Lincoln, Nebraska: University of Nebraska Press, 1984.

— . "Running Toward Psychological Well-Being: Special Considerations for the Female Client." In *Running Therapy and Psychology,* eds. M. Sachs and G. Buffone. Lincoln, Nebraska: University of Nebraska Press, 1984.

— . "Running Strategies for Women and Men." In *Running Therapy and Psychology,* eds. M. Sachs and G. Buffone. Lincoln, Nebraska: University of Nebraska Press, 1984.

Berger, Bonnie G. and David R. Owen. "Mood Alteration with Swimming—Swimmers Really Do 'Feel Better.' " In *Psychosomatic Medicine* 45: 425–433, 1983.

Brownell, Kelly D. and Albert J. Stunkard. "Physical Activity in the Development and Control of Obesity." In *Obesity*, ed. A. J. Stunkard. Philadelphia: W. B. Saunders, 1980.

Combes, Laura and Bill Reynolds. *Winning Women's Bodybuilding*. Chicago: Contemporary Books, Inc., 1983.

Darden, Ellington. *The Nautilus Woman*. New York: Simon & Schuster (Fireside), 1983.

Falls, Harold B., Ann M. Baylor, and Rod K. Dishman. *Essentials of Fitness*. Philadelphia: Saunders College/Holt, Rinehart and Winston, 1980.

Jeffrey, D. Balfour and Nancy Lemnitzer. "Diet, Exercise, Obesity, and Related Health Problems: A Macro-Environmental Analysis." In *Advances in Behavioral Medicine,* eds. J. Ferguson and B. Taylor. Holliswood, New York: Spectrum, 1983.

Katch, Frank I., and William D. McArdle. *Nutrition, Weight Control, and Exercise*. Boston: Houghton Mifflin Company, 1977.

Olinekova, Gayle. *Go for It!* New York: Simon & Schuster (Fireside), 1982.

Sharkey, Brian J. *Physiology of Fitness*. Champaign, Illinois: Human Kinetics Publishers, 1979.

Stokes, Roberta, and D. Delzingro Farls. *Fitness Everyone!* Winston-Salem, North Carolina: Hunter Textbooks Inc., 1983.

Thompson, J. Kevin, et al. "Exercise and Obesity: Etiology, Physiology, and Intervention." *Psychological Bulletin* 91: 55–79, 1982.

Wood, Peter. *California Diet and Exercise Program*. Mountain View, California: Anderson World Books, Inc., 1982.

About the Author

Bonnie G. Berger earned her Ed.D. in physical education from Columbia University. She is a full professor at Brooklyn College of the City University of New York where she has taught for the past twelve years. She also has been a member of the faculty of Dalhousie University in Nova Scotia, at Geneseo College of the State University of New York, at Queens College of the City University of New York, and has taught physical education in the public schools. She is at present director of the Sport Psychology Laboratory at Brooklyn College and supervises the Master of Science Degree in Physical Education, with a specialization in Sport Psychology. Dr. Berger has received numerous research awards to investigate the relationship between exercise, mood, and stress reduction and has exercised regularly all of her life. She resides in New York City.